Coping with Neurologic Problems Proficiently

SECOND EDITION
NURSING84 BOOKS™
SPRINGHOUSE CORPORATION
SPRINGHOUSE, PENNSYLVANIA

NURSING84 BOOKS™

NEW NURSING SKILLBOOK™ SERIES
Giving Emergency Care Competently
Monitoring Fluid and Electrolytes Precisely
Assessing Vital Functions Accurately
Coping with Neurologic Problems Proficiently
Reading EKGs Correctly
Combatting Cardiovascular Diseases Skillfully

NURSING PHOTOBOOK™ SERIES
Providing Respiratory Care
Managing I.V. Therapy
Dealing with Emergencies
Giving Medications
Assessing Your Patients
Using Monitors
Providing Early Mobility
Giving Cardiac Care
Performing GI Procedures
Implementing Urologic Procedures
Controlling Infection
Ensuring Intensive Care
Coping with Neurologic Disorders
Caring for Surgical Patients
Working with Orthopedic Patients
Nursing Pediatric Patients
Helping Geriatric Patients
Attending Ob/Gyn Patients
Aiding Ambulatory Patients
Carrying Out Special Procedures

NURSE'S REFERENCE LIBRARY®
Diseases
Diagnostics
Drugs
Assessment
Procedures
Definitions
Practices

Nursing84 DRUG HANDBOOK™

NURSING NOW™
Shock
Hypertension

NURSE'S CLINICAL LIBRARY™
Cardiovascular Disorders
Respiratory Disorders

Coping with Neurologic Problems Proficiently

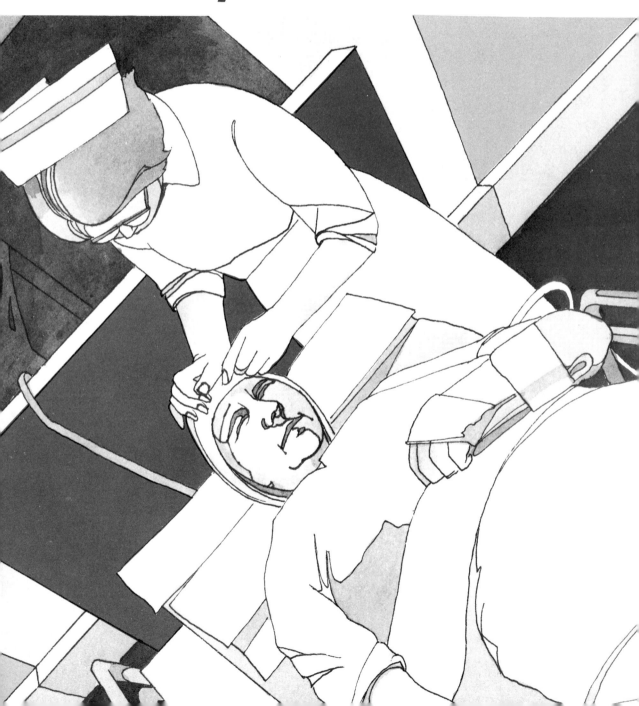

NEW NURSING SKILLBOOK™
Series
EDITORIAL PROJECT
  DIRECTOR
Jean Robinson

CLINICAL DIRECTOR
Barbara McVan, RN

ART DIRECTOR
Lisa A. Gilde

PROJECT MANAGER
Susan Rossi Williams

**Springhouse Corporation
Book Division**
CHAIRMAN
Eugene W. Jackson

PRESIDENT
Daniel L. Cheney

VICE-PRESIDENT AND
  DIRECTOR
Timothy B. King

VICE-PRESIDENT, BOOK
  OPERATIONS
Thomas A. Temple

VICE-PRESIDENT, PRODUCTION
  AND PURCHASING
Bacil Guiley

RESEARCH DIRECTOR
Elizabeth O'Brien

Staff for this edition:
BOOK EDITOR: Patricia R. Urosevich
CLINICAL EDITOR: Barbara McVan, RN
ASSISTANT EDITOR: Jo Lennon
DESIGNER: Scott M. Stephens
COPY SUPERVISOR: David R. Moreau
COPY EDITOR: Diane M. Labus
EDITORIAL ASSISTANTS: Lynn C. Borders, Ellen Johnson, Cindy O'Connell
ART PRODUCTION MANAGER: Robert Perry
ARTISTS: Diane Fox, Donald G. Knauss, Sandra Sanders, Louise Stamper, Thom
  Staudenmayer, Joan Walsh, Robert Walsh
TYPOGRAPHY MANAGER: David C. Kosten
TYPOGRAPHY ASSISTANTS: Janice Haber, Ethel Halle, Diane Paluba,
  Nancy Wirs
PRODUCTION MANAGER: Wilbur D. Davidson
COVER: Brain scan courtesy of Henry Shankin, Episcopal Hospital, Philadelphia
COVER PHOTO: Paul A. Cohen

Clinical consultant for this edition:
Vickie W. Matus, RN, BSN, MSN, CCRN, CNRN, *Neurosurgical Nurse Clinician, Mt.
  Sinai Hospital, New York*

Staff for first edition:
BOOK EDITOR: Jean Robinson
CLINICAL EDITOR: Mary Gyetvan, RN, BSEd
MARGINALIA EDITOR: Sanford Robinson
COPY EDITOR: Patricia Hamilton
RESEARCHER AND INDEXER: Vonda Heller
PRODUCTION MANAGER: Bernard Haas
TYPOGRAPHY MANAGER: David C. Kosten
PRODUCTION ASSISTANTS: Betty Mancini, Diane Paluba
ARTISTS: Bill Baker, Jamie Eisman, Robert Jackson, Kim Milnazic, Robert H.
  Renn, Sandra Simms, Carol Smith
Divider Art by Jack Freas

Clinical consultants for first edition:
Barbara Krajewski, RN, *Intensive Care Unit, Crozer-Chester Medical Center,
  Chester, Pa.*
John K. Wiley, MD, *Neurosurgeon, Assistant Clinical Professor of Surgery, Wright
  State University, School of Medicine, Dayton, Ohio*

First edition published 1978
Second edition, 1984

Library of Congress Cataloging in Publication Data

Main entry under title:

Coping with neurologic problems proficiently.
  (New Nursing Skillbook)
  "Nursing84 books."
  Bibliography: p.
  Includes index.
  1. Neurological nursing. I. Series. [DNLM: 1. Nervous
system diseases—Nursing.   WY 160 C7834]
RC350.5.C66 1984   616.8   83-20067
ISBN 0-916730-64-6

Contents

Dealing with other acute neurologic diseases

Contributors

Kathleen A. Breunig, formerly a nurse clinician in neurosurgical nursing at Madison (Wis.) General Hospital, is a graduate student at the University of Washington, Seattle. She graduated from Madison General Hospital School of Nursing and received a BSN degree from the University of Wisconsin. She's a member of the American Nurses' Association and the American Association of Neuroscience Nurses.

Lovena L. Haumann, instructor and level I coordinator at Trenton (N.J.) State College, is also a graduate of Trenton State College. She has a diploma from St. Francis Medical Center School of Nursing, Trenton, and an MA degree from New York University, where she's a PhD candidate. Ms. Haumann is a member of the American Nurses' Association and the New Jersey State Nurses' Association.

Norma M. Isaacs, who has a BN degree from McGill University, Montreal, is an operating room coordinator at Montreal Neurological Hospital. She's a member of the Canadian Nurses Association, Canadian Association of Neurological and Neurosurgical Nurses, American Association of Neuroscience Nurses, and the World Federation of Neurosurgical Nurses.

Barbara Krajewski, one of the advisors on this book, is a staff nurse in the intensive care unit at Crozer-Chester Medical Center, Chester, Pennsylvania. She graduated from Pennsylvania Hospital School of Nursing, Philadelphia, and completed a postgraduate course at the Montreal Neurological Institute. As a member of the American Association of Neuroscience Nurses, she serves on their Editorial Board and is president of the Philadelphia Chapter.

Vickie White Matus, an advisor on this edition, is a neurosurgical nurse clinician at Mt. Sinai Hospital, New York. She earned a BSN degree from Indiana University, Bloomington, and an MSN degree from the University of Cincinnati. She's a member of the American Association of Neuroscience Nurses, American Association of Critical-Care Nurses, and the Society of Critical Care Medicine.

Carol L. Mayberry has BS and MS degrees from Boston University, where she's a nurse clinician/clinical specialist at University Hospital. She's a member of the American Congress of Rehabilitation Medicine.

Marilyn Pires has an MS degree from Boston University, where she's a rehabilitation clinical nurse specialist at University Hospital. She graduated from the Samuel Merritt Hospital School of Nursing in Oakland, California, and earned a BSN degree from the University of Washington, Seattle. She's a member of the Association of Rehabilitation Nurses and the American Nurses' Association.

Kathleen Redelman is a research nurse at Indiana Neurosurgical Group, Indianapolis. She earned a BS degree from Indiana University, and is a member of the American Association of Neuroscience Nurses and the American Board of Neurosurgical Nursing.

Marilyn M. Ricci is a clinical nurse specialist at the Barrow Neurological Institute of St. Joseph's Hospital and Medical Center in Phoenix, Arizona, and an assistant professor at Arizona State University, Tempe. She graduated from State University of New York at Plattsburgh with a BS degree and earned her MS degree from Texas Woman's University, Denton. She's a member of the American Association of Neuroscience Nurses, the American Association of Critical-Care Nurses, and the American Nurses' Association.

Sharon C. Sell, a graduate of Presbyterian Hospital, Pittsburgh, is head nurse in neurosurgery at the Presbyterian University Hospital. She earned her BA degree from the University of Pittsburgh and is a member of the American Association of Neuroscience Nurses.

Nancy Swift-Bandini is a nurse in the Neurosurgical Intensive Care Unit at Hahnemann University Hospital, Philadelphia. Prior to this, she did postgraduate work in neurology and neurosurgery at National Hospital, London. She's a member of the American Association of Neuroscience Nurses and author of a book on neurological nursing.

Advisory Board

Foreword

Why have we taken the time to update this Skillbook on neurologic nursing? Consider what it offers, and you'll discover the answer. Written and revised by expert nurse clinicians—in the style of *Nursing* magazine—this Skillbook provides you with helpful, practical advice for coping with neurologic problems. What's more, these guidelines will prove valuable no matter where you work—in a general medical/surgical unit, in the emergency department, or in the ICU.

The major portion of this New Nursing Skillbook focuses on the nursing care you'll give patients with acute neurologic diseases and injuries. However, you'll find a section on chronic neurologic problems—and their care—in the Appendices. As before, this fully updated Skillbook is well illustrated, so you can better understand the basics of neurologic nursing. It's been checked and double-checked by experts to ensure accuracy and currentness.

The detailed instructions you'll find in this second edition are particularly valuable at a time when so many new techniques, potent medications, and original approaches for therapy are being used. The authors emphasize the importance of a team approach to neurologic nursing, because the wealth of scientific medical knowledge is now so great that one branch of health-care specialists can't encompass it all. They explain how to coordinate your activities with those of other team members, to bring each patient the specialized care he needs for optimal recovery.

As you examine the contents of this New Nursing Skillbook, you'll discover that—with one exception—each section discusses a different neurologic problem. The first section, however, was specially designed by the editors and artists to give you the foundation you need to understand neurologic nursing. To see what I mean by this, just turn to Chapter 1. Not only has the author reviewed the basics of the nervous system with you, but she's related those basics to the patients you may see in your unit.

In Chapter 2, you'll learn how to do a thorough neurologic assessment. Later you'll find out how to prepare your patient for the diagnostic tests he may undergo, by studying the *Nurses' Guide to Neurologic Diagnostic Tests* in the Appendices.

Like every other Skillbook, this one is packed with varied case histories, practical nursing tips, how-to-do-it photos, and patient-teaching aids.

You'll also find other helpful features throughout this book, such as the one on how to care for a patient who's immobilized and the section on monitoring intracranial pressure.

Understanding the basics and knowing the skills aren't enough when you're caring for a patient with a neurologic problem. You must also have compassion, because of all problems, these are among the most devastating. Not all patients can hope for a full recovery, even with all the medical advances made recently. These patients and their families need strong emotional support and reassurance. And you, the health-team professional they see most, must give it. By advising how to live with or compensate for a neurologic deficit, you help your patient get the best from life.

I think you'll find help in this New Nursing Skillbook for complete care of each patient. Surely, that should be your goal in neurologic nursing, because nothing less is truly adequate.

Read each chapter thoroughly; then refer back to each section as needed. Doing so will improve your skills in this specialty, and your patients will benefit.

—AGNES M. MARSHALL,
Neurosurgical Nurse Consultant
Albuquerque, New Mexico

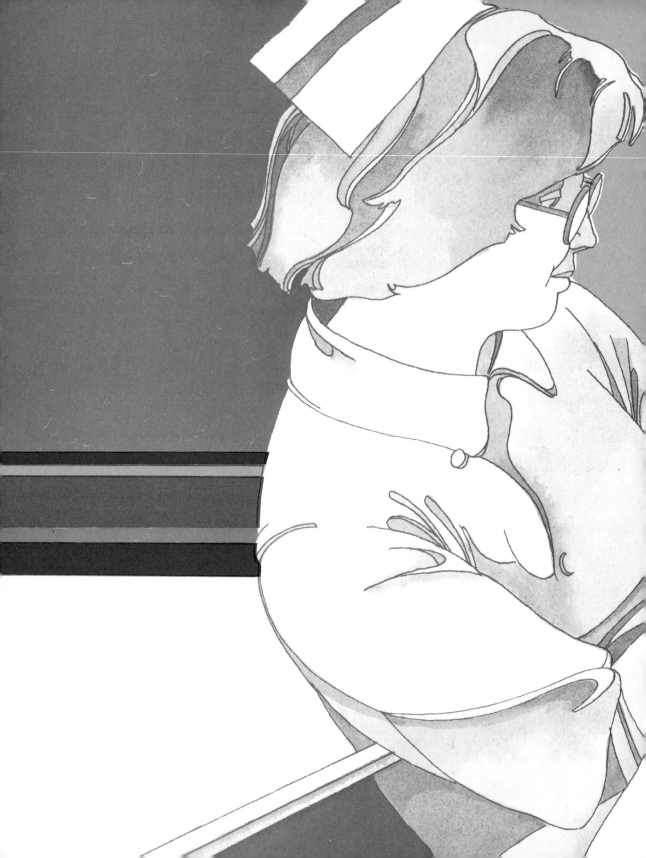

UNDERSTANDING NEUROLOGIC BASICS

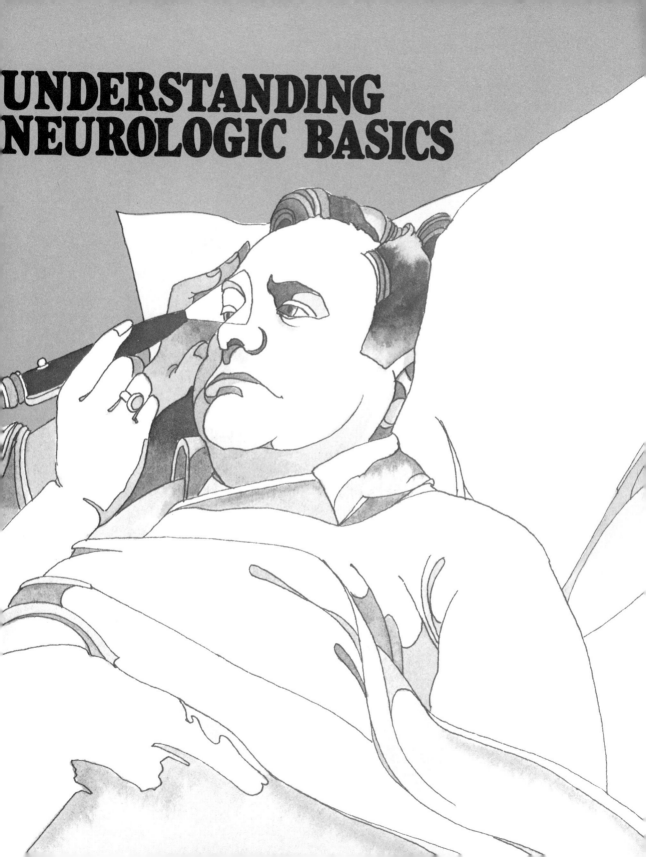

Besides the skull and vertebrae, how is the central nervous system protected?

If your patient has Parkinson's disease, which brain structure would you expect to be disturbed?

What pupillary reaction may indicate a deteriorating neurologic status?

Suppose your patient sustained an injury to the anterior portion of the frontal lobe. What are the implications and physical limitations of such an injury?

What kind of motor function can you expect from a patient with a cerebellum injury?

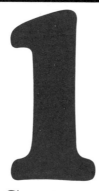

The Nervous System
Understanding how it works

BY LOVENA L. HAUMANN, RN, MA

WHAT'S YOUR REACTION when you hear the words "anatomy and physiology of the nervous system?" Does it bring back memories of long hours of grueling study? Days in which you struggled to stay afloat in a sea of information?

If so, you probably asked yourself these questions: "How much of this is really necessary for me to know as a nurse?" "Why can't I just learn to recognize and *care* for patients with neurologic diseases and injuries?" "Why must I bother with all these *technical* details?"

Perhaps your problem was one of sorting. You had trouble sifting out those details that *would* help you give your patients quality care. That's why I'm reviewing them for you in this chapter — to refresh your memory.

To help, the Skillbook artists illustrated this material lavishly, so you'll find it easier to understand. This will enable you to grasp the rest of this book quickly — and give you a solid foundation on which to build advanced nursing skills.

Our intricate communication network

You already know the two communication systems that control the billions of cells in our bodies and integrate their func-

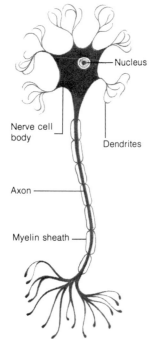

A model neuron
The basic unit of the nervous system is the nerve cell, or *neuron*. It consists of a central cell body and a number of threadlike projections of cytoplasm known as nerve fibers. These are of two types: the *axon* (conducts impulses away from the cell body) and the *dendrite* (conducts impulses to the cell body). Most neurons have multiple dendrites and a single axon.

Axons are surrounded by a white fatty substance called myelin, which insulates and protects the delicate inner fiber.

Neurons receive and transmit impulses at junctions called *synapses*, where one structure almost touches another. When information flows, the end of the axon releases a transmitting chemical that crosses the narrow cleft between the axon and the dendrite, which activates the receiving cell.

tions. These are the nervous system and the endocrine system. You also know the control center for the first of these intricate communication networks is the brain and spinal cord. We call this our central nervous system, or simply the CNS.

The nerves that extend away from this control center — to various parts of the body — are known as the peripheral nervous system (PNS). Still another subdivision is the autonomic nervous system (ANS). This regulates the functions of our internal organs and other body structures that we can't control by will.

I'll go over the central nervous system and the peripheral nervous system in greater detail later in this chapter. For an explanation of the autonomic nervous system and how it works, see pages 28 and 29.

Getting acquainted with nerve cells
Now let's talk about the two major cell types that make up the central nervous system. They are:

• *Glial cells*. These are supportive, protective cells, which are collectively called neuroglia. In Chapter 7, you'll learn that most tumors that develop within the CNS arise from neuroglia. More of these cells exist than any other type in the CNS.

• *Neuron cells*. These are highly specialized communication cells that relay impulses to, from, and within the central nervous system. As for their specific functions, there are three kinds: motor, sensory, and association. For a description of a typical neuron and how it works, see the illustration on this page.

The human computer
Housed within our cranial vault lies the most complex mechanism we know: the human brain. To properly care for your patients, you should know where each portion of the brain is located and how it operates.

For example, suppose you learn that your patient has a lesion affecting the posterior section of his left frontal lobe. Do you know what kind of signs and symptoms to expect and what to do about them?

Or suppose he's having seizures that have a definite focus in his temporal lobe? Will these differ from seizures with no definite focus?

To learn the answers to these and other questions, let's

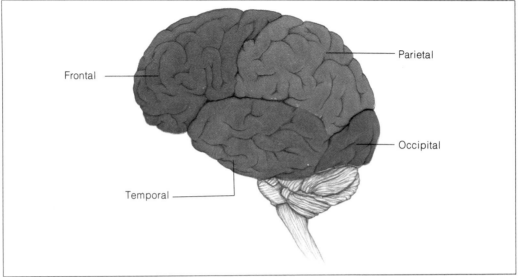

Frontal

Parietal

Occipital

Temporal

Lateral view of the brain

examine the brain's structure more closely. As you probably already know, the cerebrum — or largest part of the brain — is divided into a right and left hemisphere, separated by a longitudinal fissure. The corpus callosum, a broad band of nerve fibers, connects the cerebral hemispheres and allows for the sharing of information between them.

We call the outer layer of the cerebrum the cerebral cortex, which consists of neuron cell bodies or "gray matter." The deeper layers of each hemisphere consist of myelinated axons or "white matter," with four paired masses of gray matter areas known as the basal ganglia. When a patient has Parkinson's disease, he has a disturbance in one or more of these basal ganglia. You'll learn more about this disease and the nursing care these patients need in the Appendices.

Lobe control
To get a clear idea of how each hemisphere is further divided into lobes, study the illustration on this page. The central and limbic lobes, which are not shown on this picture, are buried deep within the fissures. The four lobes located closest to the skull are the frontal, parietal, temporal, and occipital.

What control do each of these lobes have on the body?

• *Frontal lobe*. The posterior portion of this lobe controls the patient's voluntary muscle movements. In other words, impulses originating here travel along major motor pathways to and through the spinal cord, and direct muscle movements on the opposite sides of the body.

Suppose, for example, you're managing a patient who was injured on the left side of his brain — on the posterior frontal lobe (the motor cortex). He may show partial or total paralysis on the right side of his body. If his left hemisphere is dominant, he may also lose some or all of his ability to speak. Why? Because in most cases this portion of the frontal lobe also houses the motor area for speech (Broca's area).

What about the anterior portion of the frontal lobe? This controls the patient's emotional behavior and complex intellectual activities. So your patient who was injured in this area may also show signs of agitation and confusion, and make inappropriate emotional responses.

• *Parietal lobe*. This part of the brain receives and interprets sensory impulses from the skin, muscles, joints and tendons on the opposite side of the body. Sensations processed in this lobe include: pain; heat; cold; pressure; size, shape, and texture recognition of objects; stimuli comparison for location and intensity; and body part awareness.

• *Temporal lobe*. This lobe contains the patient's centers for hearing, taste, and smell. In addition to this, the temporal lobe of the dominant hemisphere also receives and interprets sounds as words. Considering this, suppose you're caring for a patient who has a tumor involving the temporal lobe. He may suffer auditory receptive aphasia; in other words, he will hear, but won't understand the significance of the spoken word.

• *Occipital lobe*. This part of the brain receives and interprets visual stimuli. To better understand how the nerve cells transmit these impulses along the patient's visual pathways, see page 57.

• *Insula or central lobe*. As I said earlier, this lobe is buried deep within the lateral fissure. How it transmits and receives impulses is not completely understood, but the lobe seems to relate to visceral sensibility and motor activity.

• *Limbic lobe*. Although you can't see it in the illustration on page 17, the limbic lobe or system looks somewhat like a ring of brain tissue surrounding the ventricles. We sometimes hear it referred to as the visceral or emotional brain, because it's believed to link a person's higher functioning area with the more primitive areas of his brain. Damage to or malfunction of

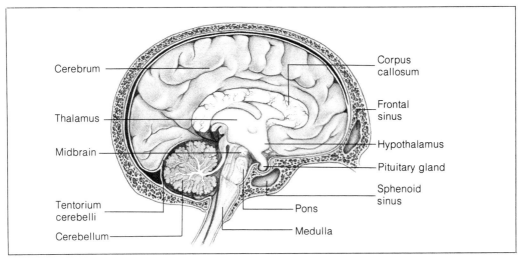

Cerebrum

Thalamus

Midbrain

Tentorium
cerebelli

Cerebellum

Corpus
callosum

Frontal
sinus

Hypothalamus

Pituitary gland

Sphenoid
sinus

Pons

Medulla

a patient's limbic system may affect his sexual behavior, emotional responses, motivation, and biological rhythms.

**Medial view of
the brain**

Getting inside

Look at the illustration on this page, which shows the brain's internal structures.

Now, direct your attention to the thalamus, what you may like to think of as a brain's sensory relay station. Just as a telegraph office relays the messages it receives to the appropriate persons, the thalamus relays incoming sensory messages to the appropriate portions of the brain. In addition, it helps distinguish between sensations that are pleasant and those that are unpleasant.

Located close to the thalamus, is the hypothalamus. It has nerve cell connections to the rest of the brain, the spinal cord, the autonomic nervous system, and the pituitary gland. When it's not functioning properly, it can affect a patient's metabolism, his body temperature, blood pressure, sleep patterns, growth, sexual maturity, and other visceral and emotional responses.

The midbrain area, plus the pons and the medulla oblongata, make up that portion of the brain we call the brain stem. Although each of these has its own special function, the brain stem unit is important for these reasons:

• It serves as a conduction pathway between the spinal cord and other parts of the brain.

CRANIAL NERVES			
	NERVE	TYPE	FUNCTIONS
I	Olfactory	Sensory	Smell
II	Optic	Sensory	Vision
III	Oculomotor	Motor	Eye movement
IV	Trochlear	Motor	Eye movement
V	Trigeminal	Motor	Chewing movements
		Sensory	Sensations of face, scalp, teeth
VI	Abducens	Motor	Eye movement
VII	Facial	Motor	Facial expressions
		Sensory	Taste; salivary and lacrimal glands
VIII	Acoustic	Sensory	Hearing; sense of balance
IX	Glossopharyngeal	Motor	Secretion of saliva; swallowing movements
		Sensory	Sensations of throat, taste
X	Vagus	Motor	Swallowing, voice production, slowing of heartbeat, and acceleration of peristalsis
		Sensory	Sensations of throat, larynx, and viscera
XI	Spinal accessory	Motor	Shoulder movements; neck rotation
XII	Hypoglossal	Motor	Tongue movements

• It houses the cell bodies for most of the cranial nerves, which you'll find discussed above.

• It — along with the thalamus and hypothalamus — contains the interlacing network of neurons and nerve fibers that make up the reticular formation. The reticular formation, as you probably know, functions as an arousal or alerting mechanism.

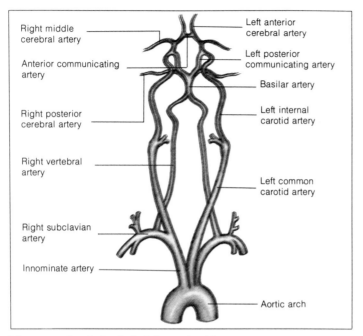

Right middle cerebral artery

Anterior communicating artery

Right posterior cerebral artery

Right vertebral artery

Right subclavian artery

Innominate artery

Left anterior cerebral artery

Left posterior communicating artery

Basilar artery

Left internal carotid artery

Left common carotid artery

Aortic arch

The brain's vascular system

You probably know that the arterial supply to the brain depends on four main arteries — the two vertebrals and the two carotids. These originate from the aortic arch or its immediate branches.

The two *vertebrals*, which are branches of the subclavians, unite to form the basilar artery. Together, they supply the *posterior* brain. The two *internal carotids* are branches of the common carotids. Branches of the internal carotid supply the anterior and middle brain.

These main vessels communicate through an arterial anastomosis at the base of the brain known as the *circle of Willis*. Its function is to provide continuity of blood circulation to the brain if any of its main vessels are interrupted.

Venous blood returns from the brain via structures called *sinuses*. These are formed by separations of the layers of the dura mater. The larger sinuses follow the course of fissures and ultimately drain into the jugular veins.

If your patient's brain is injured in this area, he may go into an irreversible coma.

In addition to these collective functions, each part of the brain stem is important for its specific reflex centers.

Nerve cell nuclei in the midbrain control various visual, auditory, and postural reflexes. For example, you'd see changes in your patient's pupillary reflexes if he had a lesion or injury that involved his midbrain.

Within the pons area, we have some of the nerve centers that control respiration rhythm. However, the critical nerve centers for a patient's cardiac, respiratory, and vasomotor functions are located in the medulla. For this reason, any serious injury to the medulla may prove fatal. (Involvement of the medulla may also affect your patient's control over his sneezing, coughing, vomiting, and swallowing.)

Now, consider the cerebellum, which you'll find just behind the brain stem. Its functions deal primarily with motor movement and equilibrium. Specifically, the cerebellum does the following:

• coordinates and refines the action of muscle groups to produce smooth, steady, precise movements

The spinal cord, nerve roots, and vertebrae

Essential to the peripheral nervous system are the 31 pairs of spinal nerves. These originate in the spinal cord and leave the vertebral canal through the *intervertebral foramina*. Spinal nerves are named by letter and number according to their point of exit:

- 8 cervical (C1-C8)
- 12 thoracic (T1-T12)
- 5 lumbar (L1-L5)
- 5 sacral (S1-S5)
- 1 coccygeal.

The cord itself usually terminates at the level of the second lumbar vertebra, so the lumbar, sacral, and coccygeal nerves must descend from their point of origin to their respective foramina. Because the end of the cord and its attached nerves resemble a horse's tail, it's called the *cauda equina*.

After leaving the vertebral column, each nerve divides into several branches or *rami*. In turn, these provide peripheral distribution characterized by extensive, but orderly, overlapping. With such extensive coverage, only minimal loss of sensory or motor function occurs if a single spinal nerve gets interrupted.

The brachial plexus and the lumbosacral plexus form a complex network of nerve fibers. They provide for further sharing and rearrangement of spinal nerve fibers.

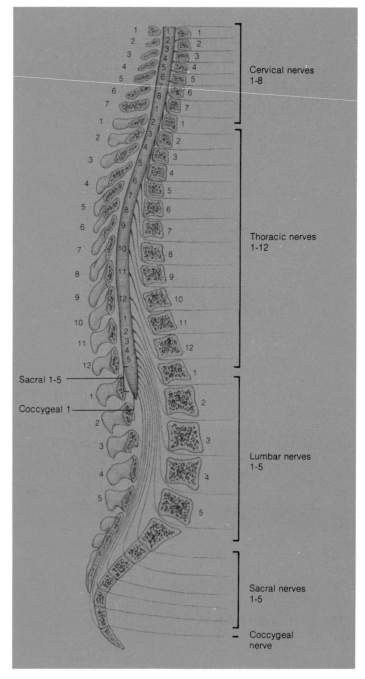

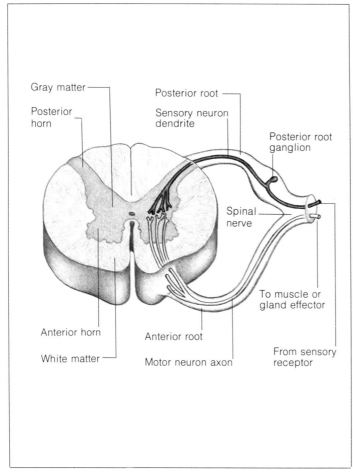

Gray matter

Posterior horn

Posterior root

Sensory neuron dendrite

Posterior root ganglion

Spinal nerve

Anterior horn

White matter

Anterior root

Motor neuron axon

To muscle or gland effector

From sensory receptor

A cross section of the spinal cord

Cross section reveals an internal mass of gray matter shaped rather like a butterfly. The gray matter is divided into areas called *horns* which consist mainly of cell bodies. Those in the *posterior* or dorsal horn serve primarily as a relay station in the process of *sensation*. Those in the *anterior* or ventral horn are essential for voluntary or reflex *motor* activity. The outer layers of the cord consist of white matter composed of thousands of myelinated nerve fibers. White matter is arranged in vertical columns which contain *tracts*, or large bundles of nerve fibers arranged in functional groups.

Looking along the horizontal axis, we see that each spinal nerve is attached to the cord by two roots:

• *Anterior* or ventral root which consists of motor (efferent) fibers leaving the cord en route to muscles and glands.

• *Posterior* or dorsal root which consists of sensory (afferent) fibers that transmit information from the sensory receptors to the spinal cord. Note that just before the posterior root joins the cord, it is marked by a swelling called the *posterior root ganglion* consisting of cell bodies of sensory neurons.

• coordinates all visual, auditory, tactile, and proprioceptive impulses with muscle activity to maintain balance and equilibrium

• maintains muscle tone.

Suppose the patient you've been caring for has an injury confined to his cerebellum. He won't be paralyzed because of it, but he probably will move jerkily and lack coordination.

How the spinal cord works

Now that we've considered the brain and how it works, let's take a close look at the spinal cord and how it relays impulses.

As you can see by the illustrations on these pages, the

A simple reflex arc

The simplest sensory-to-motor transmission path is the *reflex arc*. The classic demonstration of this is the knee-jerk reflex, elicited when you strike the tendon just below the kneecap. Here's what happens:
- The hammer strikes the tendon, which in turn stretches the quadriceps femoris muscle.
- Stretching excites the sensory nerve process, which sends an impulse to the cell body in the spinal cord. This cell then synapses with a motor neuron.
- The motor cell body sends an impulse toward a motor end-plate in the quadriceps femoris muscle. The end-plate releases the transmitting compound, *acetylcholine*, which crosses a synaptic cleft to the muscle.
- Acetylcholine then stimulates the muscle to contract.

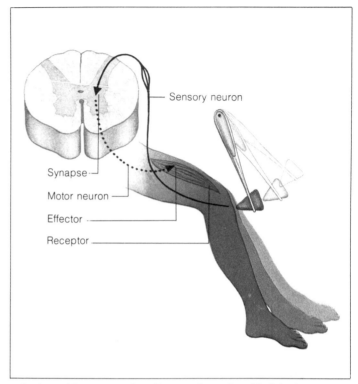

spinal cord is a somewhat flattened, oval, cylindrical structure which extends downward from the brain stem at the foramen magnum level and terminates at the second lumbar vertebra. As you no doubt know, it lies entirely within the vertebral column, which serves as its support and protection. Besides serving as a two-way conduction pathway between the brain and peripheral nervous system, it also contains the reflex centers for those activities which don't require control by the brain. (For an example of what I mean by a spinal cord reflex, see the illustration and explanation on this page.)

Now let's talk about the two-way conduction pathways I've just mentioned. If you study the picture on page 25, you'll see that these pathways consist of white matter or myelinated nerve fibers arranged in columns or funiculi. Each column contains tracts or bundles of fibers that are functionally distinct from one another. For example, some of these tracts carry sensory impulses up the spinal cord — and are called sensory tracts. And some of these tracts carry motor impulses

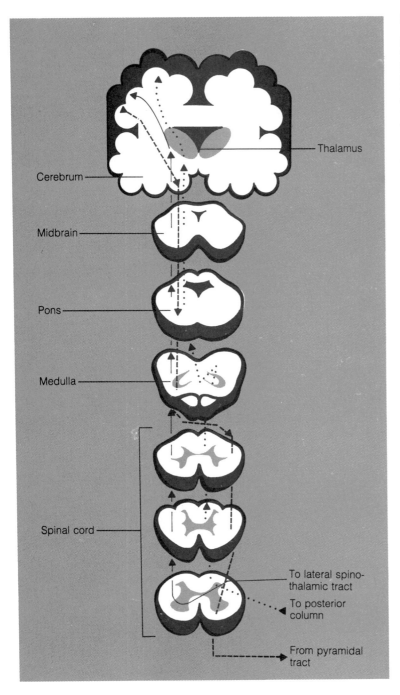

Thalamus

Cerebrum

Midbrain

Pons

Medulla

Spinal cord

To lateral spino-
thalamic tract

To posterior
column

From pyramidal
tract

How conduction pathways work

Many conduction pathways, or tracts, run through the CNS transmitting impulses. For simplicity, we have illustrated only a few of the major tracts leading to and from one side of the brain. Look closely at the positions of the tracts and the directions in which the impulses flow, paying special attention to where the fibers cross. This will help you to understand which side of the body will be affected by disease or injury at different levels and on different sides of the CNS.

• The *pyramidal tract* descends, transmitting motor impulses. Most of its fibers cross in the middle of the medulla.

• The two tracts found in the *posterior column* ascend, transmitting muscle and joint sensations of position, vibration, and pressure. These fibers also cross to the opposite side in the medulla.

• The lateral *spinothalamic tract* ascends, transmitting sensations of pain and temperature. Its fibers cross to the opposite side as they enter the cord.

down the spinal cord—and are called motor tracts.

To get a better idea of how these two-way conduction pathways work, look once more at the illustration and explanation on page 25. The description of the various tracts will help you understand why a partial transection of the spinal cord can cause loss of pain and temperature sensation on one side of the patient's body, and loss of touch, pressure sensation, voluntary movement, and position on the other side. You can also see if a patient has an injury that completely transects his cord; impulses (both sensory and motor) can no longer travel to and from his brain. This results in the loss of sensation and paralysis of all voluntary movement below the level of transection. (You'll learn more about this in Chapter 6, where spinal injuries are discussed.)

Now let's see how impulses travel over the conduction pathways. For example, how does a motor impulse traveling from the brain reach one of the patient's skeletal muscles and cause contraction? Its journey begins at an upper motor neuron in the brain, then continues to the lower motor neuron in the spinal cord. Two major categories of upper motor neurons exist—those that are part of the pyramidal system and those that are part of the extrapyramidal system:

• *Pyramidal system neurons.* These upper motor neurons originate in the motor cortex of the frontal lobe and descend through the brain's internal capsule. Most then cross the midline in the pyramids of the medulla and pass downward to the spinal cord. Impulses from these neurons control the fine, skilled movements of skeletal muscles.

• *Extrapyramidal system neurons.* These upper motor neurons also originate in the motor cortex of the frontal lobe but are mediated by such structures as the basal ganglia, thalamus, cerebellum, and reticular formation before descending to the spinal cord. Impulses from these neurons control the patient's gross motor movements and posture.

Now let's assume the impulse traveling from the upper motor neuron has reached the lower motor neuron in the patient's spinal cord. From this relay station, it travels along nerve fibers extending *out* from the cord until it reaches skeletal muscles—or effectors.

Tracking sensory impulses
But how does a sensory impulse traveling from any part of the

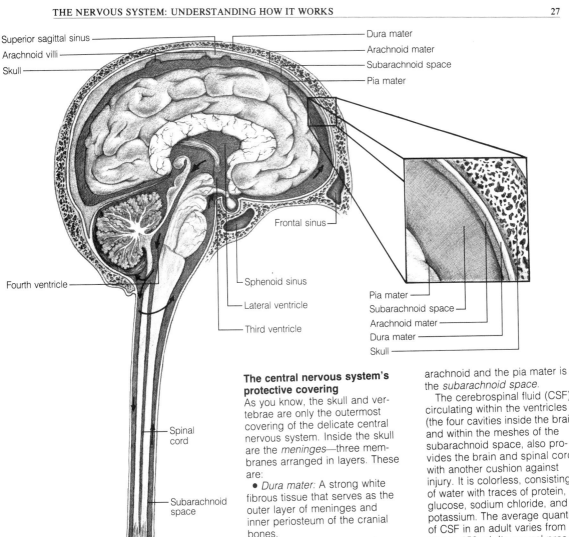

Superior sagittal sinus
Arachnoid villi
Skull
Dura mater
Arachnoid mater
Subarachnoid space
Pia mater
Frontal sinus
Sphenoid sinus
Lateral ventricle
Third ventricle
Fourth ventricle
Spinal cord
Subarachnoid space
Cauda equina
Pia mater
Subarachnoid space
Arachnoid mater
Dura mater
Skull

The central nervous system's protective covering

As you know, the skull and vertebrae are only the outermost covering of the delicate central nervous system. Inside the skull are the *meninges*—three membranes arranged in layers. These are:

• *Dura mater:* A strong white fibrous tissue that serves as the outer layer of meninges and inner periosteum of the cranial bones.

• *Arachnoid membrane:* A delicate cobwebby layer between the dura mater and the innermost layer of the meninges.

• *Pia mater:* A transparent layer that adheres to the actual surface of the brain and cord. It carries most of the brain's blood supply.

As the illustration shows, the meninges are separated by spaces. Between the dura mater and the arachnoid membrane there's a potential space called the *subdural space;* between the arachnoid and the pia mater is the *subarachnoid space.*

The cerebrospinal fluid (CSF), circulating within the ventricles (the four cavities inside the brain) and within the meshes of the subarachnoid space, also provides the brain and spinal cord with another cushion against injury. It is colorless, consisting of water with traces of protein, glucose, sodium chloride, and potassium. The average quantity of CSF in an adult varies from 100 to 150 ml. Its normal pressure is about 150 mm H_2O, or about twice that of body veins.

CSF is manufactured from the blood in capillary networks called *choroid plexuses.* Once formed, it flows from lateral to third, to fourth ventricles. Then it enters the subarachnoid spaces and is absorbed by the arachnoid villi. Eventually, it reaches the sinuses on the brain's surface where it enters into the venous blood of the brain.

How the autonomic nervous system works

The autonomic nervous system (ANS) regulates body functions that can't be controlled by will; for example, blood pressure, water balance, and digestion. It has two divisions: *sympathetic* and *parasympathetic*. The sympathetic system regulates the body's expenditure of energy, especially in times of stress. The parasympathetic system regulates the body's "domestic" functions and helps it conserve energy. Both receive their orders from the central nervous system.

Let's see how this works. The figure opposite shows how neurons for the sympathetic system are located in the part of the spinal cord that runs through the thoracic and lumbar regions. When impulses from the CNS reach these neurons, they travel along preganglionic nerve fibers to a relay station directly outside the spinal column or even more outlying. These relay stations are called ganglia. From these, postganglionic nerve fibers proceed to their destinations where they trigger the release of a catecholamine, *norepinephrine.* All postganglionic nerve fibers in the sympathetic system are called *adrenergic.*

Neurons for the parasympathetic system are located in the brain stem and the sacral segments of the spinal cord. Like sympathetic system nerve fibers, they also transmit impulses from the CNS along preganglionic nerve fibers. However, their relay stations (ganglia) are located in or near the organ involved. Here, postganglionic nerve fibers trigger the release of the neurohormone, *acetylcholine.* These neurons are *cholinergic.*

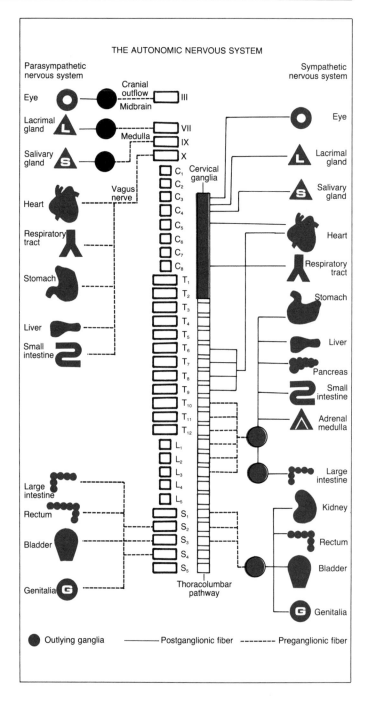

THE AUTONOMIC NERVOUS SYSTEM

Effects of autonomic nervous system		
	SYMPATHETIC	PARASYMPATHETIC
Heart	Increases rate	Decreases rate
Bronchi	Dilates	Constricts
GI tract	Decreases motility; contracts sphincters; inhibits secretions	Increases motility; relaxes sphincters; stimulates secretions
Bladder	Relaxes bladder muscle; constricts sphincter	Contracts bladder muscle; relaxes sphincter
Pupil	Dilates	Constricts
Adrenal gland	Stimulates secretion of epinephrine, norepinephrine	No significant effect

Blood vessels
  Coronary
  Skeletal muscle
  Skin and most others
	
	Dilates
	Dilates
	Constricts
		
		No significant effect
		No significant effect
		No significant effect

body reach the brain. Its journey begins at the point of stimulus and is relayed along a conduction pathway consisting of three sensory neurons. For areas supplied by spinal nerves, this relay system works as follows:

• Sensory neuron I. The receptors of this neuron set up a neural impulse in response to a stimulus. (These receptors, as you know, are the beginnings of dendrites of sensory neurons.) This impulse is then conducted along the length of the dendrite to the cell body in the dorsal root ganglion. From here, the axon conducts the impulse into the spinal cord where it synapses with the dendrites of sensory neuron II.

• Sensory neuron II. Its cell body is located in the dorsal gray horn of the cord or in the gray matter of the brain stem. The axon of this neuron conducts the impulse up to the thalamus or "sensory sorting center." For the most part, sensory messages cross before reaching the cerebral cortex, and it's usually the axon of this second neuron that crosses at some level as it ascends to the thalamus. In the thalamus, the axon of the second sensory neuron synapses with sensory neuron III.

• Sensory neuron III. The axon of this final neuron in the

relay system conveys the impulse from the thalamus to the appropriate area of the parietal lobe. It's here that perception of the sensation occurs.

What about protection?

All these wondrous and vital structures and mechanisms are not without protection. Nature has provided not one, but three ways to achieve this end. You'll find them illustrated and described in greater detail on page 27, but briefly they are:

• Bone. The skull and vertebral column provide both protection and support for delicate nervous tissue.

• Meninges (or coverings). Specifically, these coverings of the brain and cord are called the dura, the arachnoid, and the pia mater.

• Cerebrospinal fluid. This is a clear, odorless, colorless fluid that circulates around the brain and spinal cord and acts as a water jacket, providing protection.

Remember these important points when studying the nervous system:

1. Consider an understanding of brain structure and function essential to identifying and relating key signs and symptoms.

2. When a patient's temperature shows a marked change, suspect damage to the hypothalamus—the body's temperature-regulating center.

3. Be aware that any disease or injury involving a patient's cerebellum or basal ganglia affects his coordination.

4. Test your patient's sensory-to-motor transmission pathway by checking his reflexes. If this pathway is diseased or destroyed, reflexes will be absent or exaggerated.

5. If your patient has a partial spinal cord transection, expect to find a loss of pain and temperature sensation on one side of the body, and a loss of touch, pressure sensation, voluntary movement, and position sense on the other side.

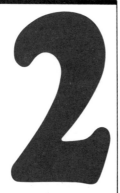

Neurologic Assessment
Keeping it ongoing

BY MARILYN M. RICCI, RN, MS, CNRN

MOST DISEASES AND INJURIES of the nervous system cause characteristic changes in function. Do you know how to recognize and evaluate these changes? You must, to do a proper assessment. Your findings — along with the results of various diagnostic tests — are important to the doctor making the diagnosis.

In some cases, what you discover during a neurologic check may be the first indication that something's gone wrong with the patient's nervous system. You may prevent dangerous complications. That's reason enough to be skilled in this area. But the patient's life may also depend on your ability.

How comprehensive an exam?
As you know, this Skillbook focuses on immediate care for acute, life-threatening situations. For that, you won't need the most extensive neurologic check possible, but one examining these five critical areas: level of consciousness, pupillary activity, motor function, sensory function, and vital signs.

Of these five, the patient's level of consciousness best indicates brain function. In most cases, it provides your first clue to a deteriorating condition.

Eye opener
Your patient's ability to open his eyes is a good test of his level of consciousness, so include this observation when you assess his condition. Note and record whether he opens his eyes as a response to sound, a direct command, or pain. If his level of consciousness is severely impaired, he may not open his eyes even in response to a painful stimulus. This may indicate a severe depression of his brain stem's arousal system. Remember however, that facial paralysis or trauma can also prevent him from opening his eyes.

Assessing level of consciousness

In upcoming chapters, we'll discuss how specific diseases and injuries can impair level of consciousness. In some way, all these disorders depress or destroy the brain stem's reticular-activating mechanism or the conduction pathways leading to and from the cerebral cortex (see Chapter 1).

By assessing level of consciousness, you learn how well (if at all) your patient perceives and responds to environmental stimuli. To elicit a response, you may have to inflict pain to get any response at all.

Eliciting verbal responses

Proper assessment of level of consciousness involves two phases: one to evaluate verbal responses, and one to evaluate motor responses.

Let's start with the first phase, in which you evaluate your patient's ability to respond verbally. Observe him closely, and ask yourself these questions:

• Is he alert? Can you get his attention easily?

• Does he seem more lethargic or drowsy than usual? Are you having more trouble getting his attention? If he's asleep, is he hard to awaken? *Important:* Make sure your patient isn't sedated when you evaluate his response.

• Is he getting restless? For example, is he tossing and turning about more? Is he irritable?

Next, talk to him to see if he's well-oriented to his surroundings. First, ask him who he is. Can he tell you the correct month and year? Does he know he's in the hospital? Does he recognize family and friends? (If none are around, ask him to name someone who's been close to him for a long period of time.)

If your patient is becoming disoriented, you'll notice changes occuring in this order: First, he'll lose all sense of time. Then, he may be confused about where he is. Next, he may not recognize family members or friends. And finally, he'll stop responding to his name and won't be able to tell you who he is.

Important: Does your patient seem confused? Keep in mind that the reason may be other than neurologic. For example, he may not fully understand the language you're speaking; he may be confused about frequent transfers within the hospital; or he may be suffering sensory deprivation.

When you evaluate your patient's verbal responses, note whether or not his replies were comprehensible. If he made only moaning or groaning sounds, specify this in your notes. If he made no response, write "no verbal response." Leaving a space blank may suggest you forgot to check everything.

Eliciting motor responses

Now let's discuss the second phase in assessing level of consciousness: evaluating motor responses. First, see if your patient responds to simple verbal or written commands. For example, ask him to open his eyes, stick out his tongue, hold up his arms, or squeeze and release your fingers.

Important: When you're testing his extremities, be sure to include both sides of his body. The best response in the arms is the clearest indicator of consciousness level.

Did he respond in some way? If so, document exactly how — and to which commands — on the patient's progress notes.

If your patient doesn't respond to your commands, you will have to resort to unpleasant or painful stimuli. Always try patting him on the arm before you use a painful stimulus, however. This may be enough to cause an immediate response.

Nothing yet? Then, apply a painful stimulus, using the least amount necessary to elicit a response. Probably the safest way to do this: Exert pressure on the patient's fingernail bed with a pencil or pen.

If he still doesn't respond, apply pressure to his supraorbital notch. You'll find out exactly how to do this on this page. (Refer to page 34 for motor responses to this stimulus.)

Caution: Never pinch the patient's skin when you use any of these measures; you may bruise him. Also, if friends or family members are present, be sure to explain what you're doing.

Evaluating responses

How do you evaluate your patient's responses to painful stimuli? Remember that his responses will grow less purposeful as his condition deteriorates. At first, he'll probably sense where you're applying the stimulus and respond by reaching up to remove it, or by trying to withdraw from it.

However, as his condition worsens, he may no longer localize pain and respond to it in a purposeful way. Instead, he may have a decorticate response, one in which his arms are

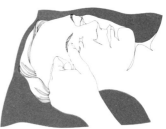

A painful stimulus
If you must apply a painful stimulus to elicit a response from your patient, apply light to moderate pressure with your thumb to the bony ridge under his eyebrow. Can your patient localize pain? If he can, he'll reach up towards the stimulus. Caution: Take care not to injure your patient's eye.

Motor responses to pain

When you apply a painful stimulus to your unconscious patient's supraorbital notch, he'll respond in one of these ways:

LOCALIZING PAIN (Fig. 1): An appropriate response is to reach up above shoulder level toward the stimulus. Remember, a focal motor deficit such as hemiplegia may prevent a bilateral response.

As brain stem involvement increases, your patient may respond by assuming one of the following postures. Each one shows more advanced deterioration.

DECORTICATE POSTURING (Fig. 2): One or both arms in full flexion on the chest. Legs may be stiffly extended.

DECEREBRATE POSTURING (Fig. 3): One or both arms stiffly extended. Possible extension of the legs.

FLACCID (Fig. 4): No motor response in any extremity. An extremely ominous sign.

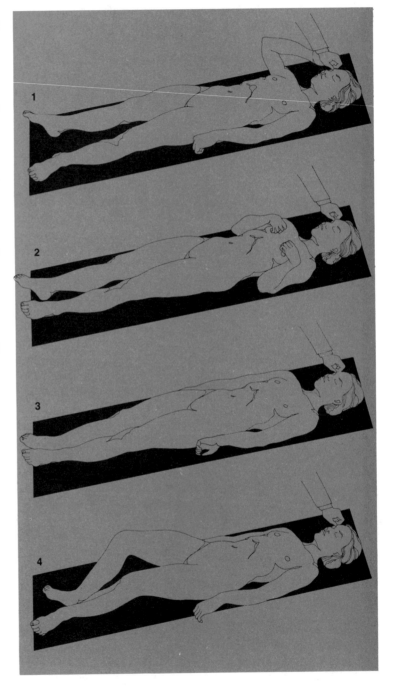

sharply flexed on his chest and his legs are stiffly extended. Next he'll have a decerebrate response, one in which all four limbs are stiffly extended. In some cases, fragments or combinations of these responses occur or, when the patient's condition is very grave, no response may occur. (For a more complete description of these responses and how they relate to the location of the lesion, see the opposite page.)

Documenting level of consciousness

What's the proper way to describe your patient's level of consciousness, once you've evaluated it? Do you write one-word terms such as "lethargic," "stuporous," or "semicomatose?" Frankly, I think such terms are too vague and easily misinterpreted. Better record only specific facts. For example, write exactly what stimulus you used, where you applied it, how much pressure you needed to elicit a response, and how the patient responded. Describe the response as clearly as possible. Don't write something like "patient jerked and changed position"; instead, write something like "patient grimaced and flexed left toes in response to fingernail pressure."

How to assess pupillary activity

Now, let's consider how to assess your patient's pupillary activity. As you may recall from Chapter 1, pupillary constriction is controlled by the oculomotor or third cranial nerve, which arises from the brain stem. Because of this, any pupillary changes that occur may indicate third cranial nerve involvement and possible brain stem damage. However, other conditions may be responsible for pupil abnormalities: For example, the patient may have suffered a serious eye injury, or he may be taking drugs.

To properly assess your patient's pupillary activity, you must closely observe the size and shape of his pupils, whether or not they're equal, and how they react to light.

Here's how. Observe the appearance of his pupils by holding his eyelids open and inspecting his pupils for size, shape, and equality. Normal pupils are round, usually at a midposition, and have a diameter ranging from 1.5 to 6 millimeters. When you're doing a neurologic check, be specific about the size when you document it in your notes (see page 36). Don't write vague terms like "constricted," "pinpoint," or "di-

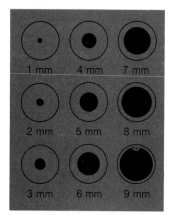

Grading pupils
Monitoring your patient's pupillary activity is an important part of neurologic nursing care. But how do you compare your findings at, say, 4 p.m. with those of another nurse at 2 p.m.? To do so, you need to know something more specific than "right pupil more dilated than left."

To help you and other health-team members compare findings, here's a way to evaluate pupil sizes precisely: Put a scale showing sizes in millimeters at the top of the patient's flow chart. Then, each nurse can compare pupillary changes against an absolute, and identical, frame of reference.

lated." If you do, others may have a hard time making a comparison later in case of changes.

Remember, your patient's pupil size may vary considerably from another patient's and still be normal. He may even have normally *unequal* pupils. To evaluate his pupil size properly, try to find out what's normal for *him* and record that information in his patient history.

Next, assess how your patient's pupils react to light. *Darken his room and use a small, bright penlight.* To test direct light reflex, hold each eyelid open in turn, keeping the opposite eye covered. Now, move the light toward the patient from the side. Shine it directly into his eye, which should cause his pupil to constrict promptly. Make a note of your findings.

Now test his consensual light reflex. To do this, hold both eyelids open, but shine the light into one eye only. *Watch the other one.* Does that pupil constrict also? It should, indicating intact connections between the brain stem areas regulating pupil constriction.

Important: Be sure to document any unusual eye movements: for example, a deviation from midline, or absence of conjugate gaze. These abnormalities may mean cranial-nerve damage.

Interpreting your findings
Now that you've tested your patient's pupillary reflexes, how do you interpret your findings? Watch for a sluggish reaction to light and report it promptly. In many cases, it's an early warning that the patient's condition is deteriorating. Unequal pupil sizes may indicate his parasympathetic and sympathetic nervous systems aren't working together as they should. If your patient has a dilated and nonreactive pupil on only one side, *call the doctor immediately.* This could be from increased intracranial pressure, or ipsilateral oculomotor nerve compression from tumor or injury. (For further information on how to assess and interpret pupillary activity, see page 90.)

How to assess motor function
Damage to almost any part of your patient's nervous system can affect his ability to move. If you think back to Chapter 1, you'll probably recall how motor function is controlled by certain areas in the brain. From these areas, impulses travel along extensive motor pathways. When any part of this com-

plicated network gets damaged by disease or injury, motor function may be lost or impaired. As I explain how to assess your patient's motor function, refer to the chart on this page. It'll give you some clues that may indicate the location of the lesion. Six things to observe closely when you assess motor functioning are:

- muscle strength
- muscle tone
- posture
- muscle coordination
- reflexes
- abnormal movements, if any exist.

I'll tell you exactly how to do this in the following paragraphs. But first, I want to offer you some general guidelines that apply to all motor-function assessments.

Don't miss these important checks

Keep in mind that you're not only noting the presence of movement (and its quality); you're also noting the absence of movement, as well. When movement exists, record the best response *in each extremity*. Note any weakness the patient shows. Compare each motor response in an extremity to its

Locating lesions			
Your assessment of your patient's motor activity may help to pinpoint the site of his lesion. Refer to this chart. It shows how lesion sites are related to specific motor problems you may see in your patient.			
	LOWER MOTOR NEURON	PYRAMIDAL TRACT	EXTRAPYRAMIDAL TRACT
Major effect	Flaccid paralysis	Spastic paralysis with hyperactive reflexes	No paralysis Altered muscle tone and abnormal movements
Muscle appearance	Atrophy Small muscular contractions	Mild atrophy from disuse	Tremor when at rest
Muscle tone	Decreased	Increased	Increased
Muscle strength	Decreased or absent	Decreased or absent	Normal
Coordination	Absent or poor	Absent or poor	Slowed

Testing muscle strength
1. Place your patient's leg with knee flexed and foot resting on the bed, as shown here. Instruct him to keep his foot down as you try to extend his leg.
2. Support his knee as shown in the illustration. Instruct him to straighten his leg as you apply resistance.
   Evaluate and document your patient's performance.
Incorporate your assessment in his care plan.

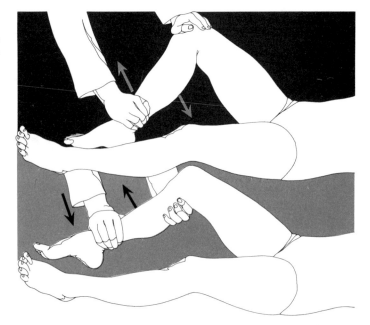

counterpart on the opposite side of the body. If you notice any change from the last neurologic check, describe it exactly. *Important:* Before you evaluate your findings, always consider other conditions that may affect your patient's motor responses: his age, arthritis, or unrelated disease or injury.

Testing the patient's muscle strength
To assess your patient's muscle strength, test it against your own muscle resistance, then against the pull of gravity.

If your patient can respond to commands, complete these tests for muscle strength:

• Test grip in both hands at the same time. Extend your hands and ask the patient to squeeze your fingers as hard as he can. Compare grip strength and document your findings.

• Test arm strength by asking the patient to close his eyes and hold his arms straight out in front of him with palms up. See if he can maintain this position for 20 to 30 seconds. If one arm drifts downward or turns inward, that may indicate hemiparesis. Document what you observe.

• Test flexion and extension strength in your patient's extremities by having him push and pull against your resistance. One way to do this: Stand in front of him and extend your

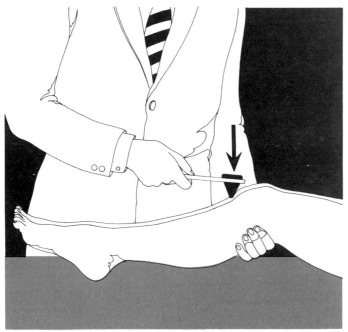

Patellar reflex — "Knee jerk"
Here's an example of a deep tendon reflex. To elicit this reflex when your patient's lying down, place your hand under his knee to raise and flex it. Then tap his patellar tendon just below the knee with a reflex hammer. If he responds normally, his leg will extend.

hands. Then ask him to push and pull against your hands. Does he show weakness? If so, is the weakness equal in both arms? Document your findings. Follow a similar procedure to test his legs (see illustration on opposite page).

When you document, use terms like "normal power," "mild weakness," or "severe weakness," since you obviously can't be as specific as you are when you measure pupillary activity.

What about the patient who can't follow commands because of a language barrier or decreased level of consciousness? First, observe his spontaneous movements and note how strong they seem. Then, if necessary, apply painful stimuli. If you get a withdrawal response from each limb, make comparisons in strength and document them.

Testing your patient's muscle tone
To properly assess your patient's muscle tone, you'll flex and extend his limbs on both sides and see how well he resists your movements. Increased resistance (for example, muscle rigidity or spasticity) means increased muscle tone. Decreased resistance (for example, limpness or flaccidity) means decreased muscle tone. Be sure to document findings.

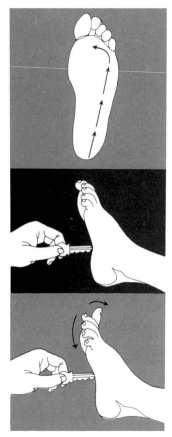

Plantar reflex
Stroke the lateral aspect of the
sole of your patient's foot (top).
The normal response is flexion of
the toes (center).
 The Babinski response is
abnormal. The great toe will
dorsiflex and the other toes fan
(bottom). This indicates an upper
motor neuron lesion.

What can this tell you about his disease or injury? Refer to
the chart of responses on page 37. It shows how a patient's
muscle tone provides clues to the site of his lesion.

Testing your patient's coordination
Any disease or injury that involves a patient's cerebellum or
basal ganglia will affect his coordination. To properly assess
your patient's hand and arm coordination, you'll use two kinds
of tests:
 • Rapid, rhythmic, alternating movements. Check each hand
separately. First, ask your patient to pat his thigh as fast as he
can. Note whether his movements seem slow or awkward.
Then, ask him to turn his hand over and back several times in
succession and evaluate his coordination during this test. Finally, ask him to touch each of his fingers with his thumb in as
rapid sequence as possible. How well does he do? Document
your findings for each limb, but keep in mind that his dominant
hand will usually perform better.
 • Point-to-point movements. Check each hand separately.
Now extend one of your hands toward him. Ask your patient
to touch first your index finger, then his nose several times in
succession. Can he do it smoothly and accurately, without
tremor? When you've evaluated his coordination with his eyes
open, ask him to repeat the test with his eyes closed. Note: If
he fails to perform the maneuver accurately with his eyes
closed, he may have lost his positioning sense.
 Once you've assessed and evaluated your patient's arm and
hand coordination, go on to the next test, which involves the
legs. The same type of test is used here; for example:
 • Rapid, rhythmic, alternating movements. Place your hands
close to the patient's feet. Now ask him to tap your hands with
the balls of his feet — doing it alternately and as quickly as
possible. Watch for slowness or awkwardness, but keep in
mind that his feet won't perform as adeptly as his hands.
 • Point-to-point movements. Check each leg separately. Ask
the patient to place a heel on his opposite knee and slide it
down his shin to his foot. Can he do this smoothly, without
tremor? Record your findings.

Assessing your patient's reflexes
You can't accurately assess and evaluate your patient's motor
functioning without checking his reflexes. In this section, I'll

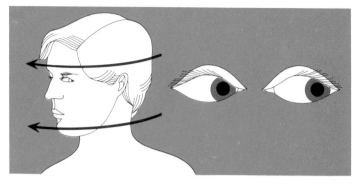

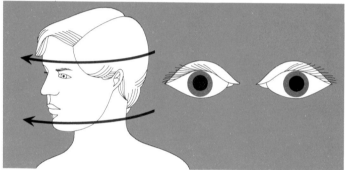

Oculocephalic reflex

How can you quickly assess brain stem function in an unconscious patient? Test his oculocephalic reflex, which is sometimes called doll's eye reflex. To test for this reflex, hold the patient's eyelids open. Then, quickly—but gently—turn his head to the right. If everything's OK, his eyes will appear to move conjugately toward the center of his body (left of his eye sockets). But if his eyes remain stationary in the center or to the right of his eye sockets, his doll's eye reflex is absent indicating a deteriorating consciousness level. Notify the doctor.

explain how to test four of the most important reflexes: blink (menace); gag and swallow; plantar; and oculocephalic.

The first two are important to check because they're protective reflexes. Checking the last two will help to determine the site of a lesion.

Because the two protective reflexes are controlled by certain cranial nerves, any disease or injury that involves these nerves will impair or eliminate the reflex. Specifically, if either or both the 5th or 7th cranial nerves are involved, the patient may have no blink reflex. If the 9th and 10th cranial nerves are involved, he may have no gag.

To test a patient's blink (menace) reflex, ask the patient to look up or hold his eyelid open. With your hand, approach his eye unexpectedly from the side or brush his eyelashes.

If his blink reflex is intact, his eye will close immediately. If it doesn't, he'll need eye care to prevent drying and irritation. Be sure to include this need on his care plan.

To test a patient's gag and swallow reflex, ask him to open

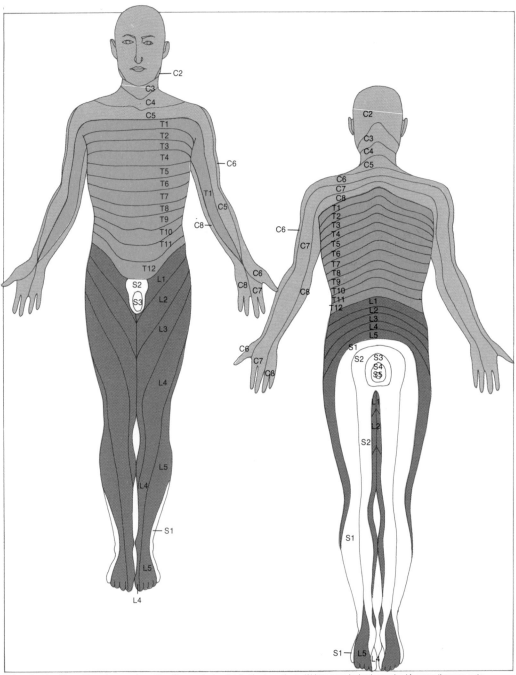

his mouth and hold down his tongue with a wooden depressor. Touch the back of his pharynx on each side with a cotton swab. If he doesn't gag or swallow spontaneously, be sure to provide suctioning as needed and watch for signs of airway obstruction. Don't give him foods or liquids orally.

For a complete explanation of how to check other important reflexes, see the illustrations on pages 40 and 41.

Check out abnormal movements

Be alert for abnormal movements when you assess motor functioning: for example, seizures and tremors. In an unconscious patient whose condition is severely deteriorated, you may also see the decorticate or decerebrate postures I explained earlier (see page 34). These postures, always ominous signs, may occur spontaneously or in response to painful stimuli.

Doing an accurate sensory assessment

Along with everything else, a complete neurologic check assesses your patient's sensory functioning. As you know, moment-to-moment sensory input enables a person to alter his responses and behavior to adapt to this environment. When disease or injury damages his sensory pathways, which are located within and outside the central nervous system, it always affects his sensory responses.

When you assess your patient's sensory functioning, check the following:

• central and peripheral vision (visual acuity and visual fields)

• hearing and ability to understand verbal communication

• superficial sensations (light touch, pain)

• deep sensations like muscle and joint pain, or sense of muscle and joint position.

Testing central and peripheral vision

Here's how to check your patient's central and peripheral vision. As you'll find out later in Chapter 3, visual abnormalities will vary, depending on the location of the lesion. One or both of the patient's eyes may be involved, and the deficit may range from blurred vision to total blindness.

To test visual acuity, ask the patient to read something aloud. Check each eye separately, covering the other with an

Dermatome chart
The illustration opposite depicts the segmental distribution of spinal nerves which transmit pain, temperature, and touch from the skin (on the front and back) to the cord. Refer to these dermatome charts when assessing your patient's sensory function. Note: Not all authorities agree on the same precise segmental levels. Other sources may show minor variations.

Visual field check

Perform this simple test if you suspect your patient has a neurologic problem affecting his peripheral vision. If results suggest a visual defect, his doctor may wish to perform a more detailed exam using special techniques.

Here's how you do it: First, position yourself so you're facing the patient, eyes level with his, about 2 feet away. Then, ask him to cover one eye without pressing on it, and to look at your eye directly opposite. Bring a pencil or another small object from the periphery into his field of vision. Do this from several directions, as illustrated. Each time, ask him to indicate when he first sees the object coming into view, and compare the extent of his vision with yours. Then repeat the test with his other eye.

Note: To test the medial field, keep the test object equidistant between you and the patient. To test the lateral field, start with the object somewhat behind the patient.

For an explanation of how intracranial lesions may affect visual pathways to produce field-cuts, see page 57.

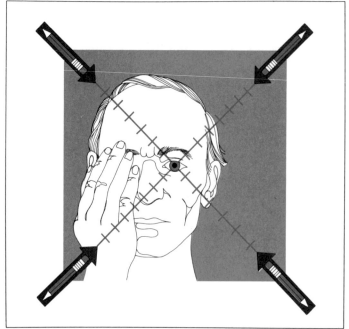

opaque card. If his vision is so poor that he can't read, ask him to count your upraised fingers or to distinguish light from dark. Use an eye chart, if the doctor wants a more precise check.

To test your patient's visual fields, use the confrontation method illustrated on this page. (Later on, the doctor will add to your findings with a more detailed exam.)

Suppose you discover from this test that your patient has some kind of visual field-cut? This can happen if his lesion affects visual pathways. Expect this patient to have some nursing care problems that'll require your immediate attention. To learn more about field-cuts and how they affect vision, see page 57.

Testing your patient's hearing and ability to understand

If your patient is conscious, but doesn't seem to hear or understand your requests, test his hearing. To do this, check one ear at a time. Occlude the ear canal with cotton. Now, standing about 2 feet away from the patient, test his un-occluded ear by softly whispering numbers. Make sure he isn't reading your lips. If he doesn't hear or understand your first attempts, whisper or speak as loud as necessary. Compare the hearing in both ears and document your findings.

In some cases, you'll sense that your patient hears but doesn't comprehend. This type of deficit is common in stroke patients and is discussed more thoroughly in Chapter 3. When you suspect a verbal comprehension deficit, take care that it's documented as such so it's not mistaken for a hearing loss.

Testing superficial sensation

Whenever you test superficial sensations, follow these guidelines:

• Pay careful attention to how well your patient perceives the stimulus and check the same area on the opposite side of body so you can make a comparison.

• When you check an extremity, begin at the furthest point and work your way toward the trunk. Make comparisons.

• Don't confine your testing to one area. Scatter stimuli over the entire body to get an accurate assessment.

• If you find an area where sensations are impaired or missing, map out its boundaries carefully. Use a dermatome chart to record your findings. You'll see an example of one you can copy for your own use on page 42. Now, here's how you do the actual tests, using the following stimuli:

• *Pain*. Ask the patient to close his eyes. Stroke his skin with the point of an open safety pin. Use the blunt end occasionally. Ask him to tell you what he feels. See if he can distinguish between "sharp" and "dull" sensations.

• *Temperature*. Ask the patient to close his eyes. Fill two test tubes with water (one hot and one cold). Touch the patient's skin with each test tube and ask him to tell you which is which.

• *Light touch*. Stroke a wisp of cotton over his skin. Ask him to tell you when he feels it.

• *Positioning*. Ask the patient to close his eyes. Then grasp the tip of one of his fingers and hold it between your thumb and index finger. Move it up and down and ask your patient to tell you in which direction it's moving. If you sense that his position sense is lost or impaired, repeat the test at his wrist and elbow. To test his legs, start with the big toe and work your way up to his knee, if necessary.

Check your patient's vital signs

No neurologic check is complete without an assessment of your patient's vital signs: respirations, temperature, blood

Danger signals
Any of these conditions in patients with neurologic problems may indicate a serious, perhaps life-threatening, situation:
• Decreasing level of consciousness
• Fixed, dilated pupil
• Decorticate or decerebrate movements
• Altered pattern of respiration.

pressure, and pulse. Of these four, his respiration will tell you the most about how his brain is functioning. The reason for this: Respirations are controlled by different areas of the brain. Anytime injury or disease affects these areas, respiratory changes may occur, as well.

Note the rate and quality of your patient's respirations, and pay careful attention to the pattern, because it can provide clues to the location of the lesion. For example, a patient who has cluster breathing may have a lesion in his upper medulla. To learn more about breathing patterns and how they relate to lesions in various parts of the brain, see the diagram on the opposite page.

As you'll discover in subsequent chapters, the patient with a neurologic problem becomes very susceptible to respiratory problems. Observe him closely and check results of lab tests necessary to assess his respirations accurately: for example, arterial blood-gas measurements and vital capacity.

What about temperature changes?
Check your patient's temperature and report any changes to the doctor. Damage to the hypothalamus, which serves as a temperature regulating center, may alter the patient's temperature so much that it'll require special nursing care. (Pay particular attention to the temperature changes accompanying spinal shock. For more information on this, read Chapter 6.)

Check blood pressure and pulse
When your check your patient's blood pressure and pulse, you'll watch him closely for signs of increased intracranial pressure (see pages 92 to 95). Specifically you'll be alert for a widening pulse pressure and a slowing pulse rate. *Caution:* These changes usually occur late, after your patient's level of consciousness has already begun to deteriorate. Call the doctor at the first sure sign of neurologic deterioration. Don't wait for the changes in blood pressure and pulse rate.

As you probably know, the signs I just mentioned are the opposite of those for hypovolemic shock, in which the blood pressure falls and the pulse rate increases. If your patient shows signs of hypovolemic shock, look for reasons other than neurologic damage. Even with head injury, a person can't lose enough blood within his cranial cavity to cause hypovolemic shock.

Abnormal respiration patterns

When caring for an unconscious patient, watch for these patterns of respiration.

PATTERN OF RESPIRATION	WHAT HAPPENS	SIGNIFICANCE
Cheyne-Stokes	Rhythmic waxing and waning of both rate and depth of respirations, alternating regularly with briefer periods of apnea.	May indicate deep cerebral or cerebellar lesions, usually bilateral. May occur with upper brain stem involvement.
Central neurogenic hyperventilation	Sustained, regular, rapid respirations, with forced inspiration and expiration.	May indicate a lesion of the low midbrain, or upper pons areas of the brain stem.
Apneustic	Prolonged inspiratory cramp with a pause at full inspiration. There may also be expiratory pauses.	May indicate a lesion of the mid- or low pons.
Cluster breathing	Clusters of irregular respirations alternating with longer periods of apnea.	May indicate a lesion of the low pons or upper medulla.
Ataxic breathing.	A completely irregular pattern with random deep and shallow respirations. Irregular pauses may also appear.	May indicate a lesion of the medulla.

Spinal cord injuries can also affect a patient's blood pressure and pulse rate. For more information on this, see Chapter 6.

Completing your assessment

To complete your neurologic assessment, check your patient's gastrointestinal activity, and observe for possible fluid and electrolyte imbalance. Also check bowel and bladder control, and listen for newly developed speech difficulties.

Document what you've found during your neurologic check, and communicate your findings to the doctor. Be sure to include the time and sequence of events when you see changes. Describe what symptoms occurred together and what changes took place since the last check.

If your patient's condition has not yet been diagnosed, the doctor will probably order several tests to help him arrive at a diagnosis. Some of these are quite arduous for the patient and will require special nursing care. The doctor will want you to prepare your patient for the tests he'll undergo and keep him from becoming frightened.

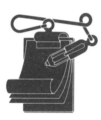

Remember these important points when assessing your patient's neurologic system:
1. Be aware that a decreased level of consciousness is usually the first clue to deteriorating brain function.
2. Consider a patient disoriented when he: loses a sense of time; is confused about his whereabouts; fails to recognize family members or friends; can't tell you who he is; or stops responding to his name.
3. When you apply painful stimulus to a patient's supraorbital notch, check for decorticate or decerebrate posturing, or flaccidity. Consider any of these responses ominous.
4. During the pupillary check, watch for a dilated and nonreactive pupil in one eye. This response may indicate increased intracranial pressure or ipsilateral oculomotor nerve compression from an injury. Report this finding to the doctor immediately.
5. Suspect a lesion affecting the visual pathways if your patient's experiencing field-cuts.

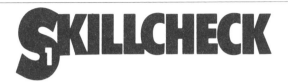

SKILLCHECK

1. Karen Dolp is a 22-year-old copywriter with amyotrophic lateral sclerosis. Reports indicate that the disease has damaged cells in the anterior gray horn of her spinal cord. Which of the following problems is she apt to have?
a) Autonomic nervous system impairment
b) Sensory loss
c) Increased spasticity of muscles
d) Paralysis

2. Mrs. Wilma Shore is admitted to the neurologic unit with a ruptured cerebral aneurysm. Tests show the lesion affects the posterior frontal lobe of her right cerebral hemisphere. What problem can you most likely expect her to have?
a) Receptive aphasia
b) Left hemiparesis or hemiplegia
c) Paraplegia
d) Right hemiparesis or hemiplegia

3. You're caring for a young woman with Guillain-Barre syndrome. She's alert, but when you check her for a gag reflex, you notice that it's missing. The doctor says her disease has affected some of her cranial nerves. Based on what you know from your assessment, which ones are they?
a) XI spinal accessory and XII hypoglossal
b) IX glossopharyngeal and X vagus
c) IV trochlear and V trigeminal
d) VI abducent and VII facial

4. When Robert Bliss had a stroke, his hypothalamus was affected. What kind of problem could this cause?
a) He may have body temperature disturbances.
b) He may have abnormal blood pressure readings.
c) He may develop a fluid and electrolyte imbalance.
d) He may have all of the above.

5. One of your patients is scheduled to have computerized axial tomography (CAT scan) of his brain without the use of a contrast medium. What will you tell him about this test?
a) Tell him that the doctor will inject a radioisotope into one of his veins, causing some temporary pain. When this is done, the technicians will pass a spe-

cial device back and forth over his head.
b) Tell him that a health-team professional will position him on a moving metal table that slides into the doughnut-shaped machine. Then he'll take an X-ray and feed the information into a computer to get a more detailed and accurate picture.
c) Tell him that the doctor will inject air or dye into his spinal canal. During the procedure, he may feel some pressure sensations. After that, a technician will ask him to roll over on his side for an X-ray.
d) Tell him that the technician will put some painless electrodes on his scalp. Then, as he rests quietly in bed, a special computer will record the electrical activity of his brain.

6. When you use painful stimuli to determine your patient's level of consciousness, which response indicates the highest level of functioning?
a) Decorticate posturing
b) Decerebrate posturing
c) Flaccid paralysis
d) Purposeful withdrawal

7. What is the most important and reliable index of your patient's neurologic status?
a) Vital signs
b) Pupillary reaction
c) Level of consciousness
d) Motor activity

8. Your patient has a positive Babinski reflex. What does this mean?
a) Lower motor neuron disease
b) Upper motor neuron disease
c) Spinothalamic tract degeneration
d) Posterior column tract degeneration

9. How can you assess your patient's superficial sensations?
a) Elicit knee-jerk response by patellar tapping.
b) Pinch his skin in different locations to elicit pain.
c) Pass a wisp of cotton over various areas of his body and note when he feels it.
d) Turn his head from side to side and note which way his eyes move.

(Answers on page 175)

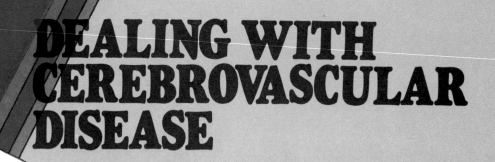

DEALING WITH CEREBROVASCULAR DISEASE

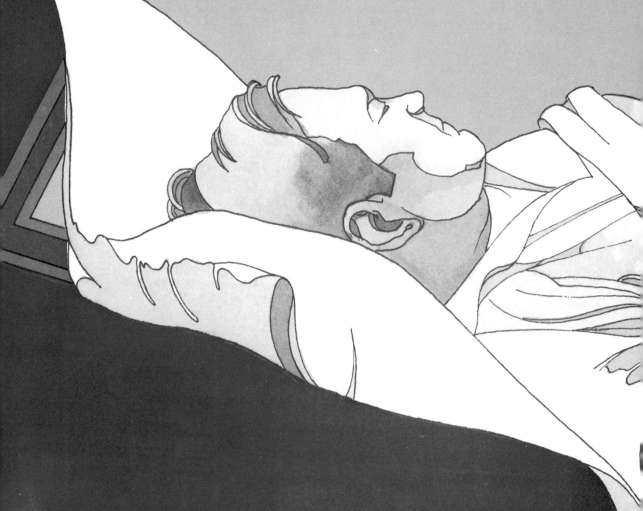

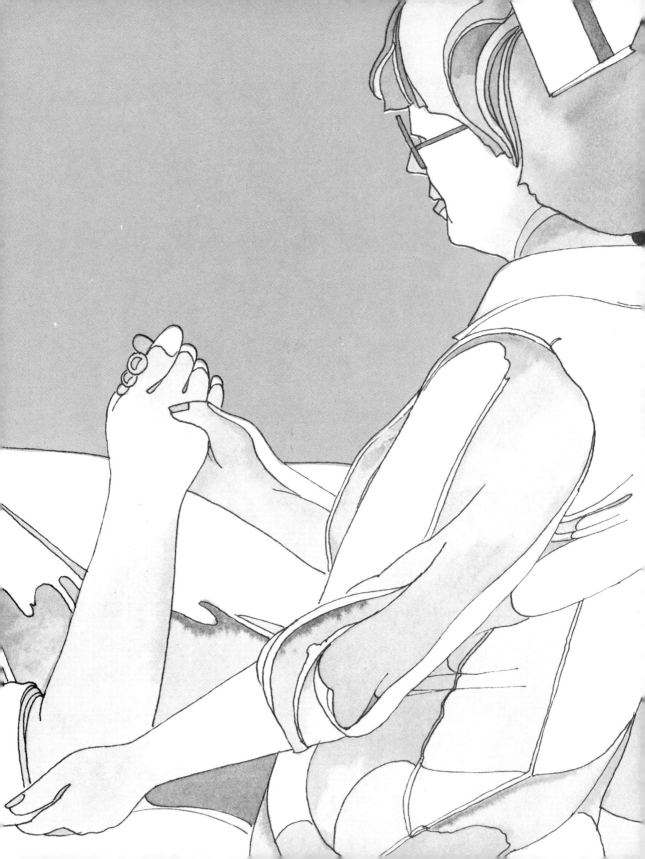

What six criteria affect how your patient
will recover from a CVA?

If your patient's suffered a CVA involving
the carotid artery, what telltale
signs and symptoms will he exhibit?

What nursing actions can you
take to improve communication with
an aphasic patient?

What life-threatening problems
frequently occur in a patient with a
cerebral aneurysm rupture?

What test generally confirms a cerebral
aneurysm rupture?

3

Cerebrovascular Accident
Providing acute care

BY KATHLEEN REDELMAN, RN, BS, CNRN

"HE'D BEEN ACTING just fine until about an hour ago," the weathered ranch hand tells you, anxiously. He's referring to his boss, 56-year-old Sam Brand, who he's just driven 30 miles to the emergency department of the hospital where you work.

According to the worried ranch hand, Mr. Brand had been "going over papers" in his office. "Then suddenly, the boys and me spotted him coming up to the corral fence, kind of dragging himself on his right side."

You look closely at the well-tanned Mr. Brand, who's awake and seems alert, despite gross neurologic deficits. He tries to talk, but his speech is so slurred you can't understand him easily. His right arm has slipped off the examining table, without his noticing, and he lacks spontaneous control of his right leg. His vital signs are as follows: blood pressure 160/100, temperature 98.6° F. (37.0° C.), pulse 90 and regular, and respirations 18, regular and unlabored.

What do you do now, while you're waiting for the doctor to come? You're aware that Mr. Brand may have suffered a cerebrovascular accident (CVA), or what we usually refer to as a stroke. Do you know what kind of emergency care he may need? How can you determine the exact extent of his

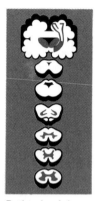

Pathophysiology
A cerebrovascular accident (CVA) occurs when there's a decrease in blood supply to a portion of the brain. As you know, interrupted or diminished oxygen supply may cause serious damage to neurons, with possible necrosis, unless normal circulation is restored within a few minutes.

The most common causes of CVA are:
• thrombosis
• embolus
• hemorrhage (see next page).

In a thrombotic stroke, the cerebral artery lumen becomes occluded, usually because of atherosclerosis. This is the most common type of cerebrovascular disease, generally occurring in the middle-late years.

An embolism, however, can occur at any age. When an embolus reaches the cerebral vasculature, it may lodge at a narrowed portion of an artery, thereby cutting off circulation. Most susceptible to emboli are patients who have:
• mural thrombi from athero-sclerotic or rheumatic heart disease
• thrombi secondary to myocardial infarction
• recently undergone cardiac surgery.

neurologic deficits? What problems is he likely to have during his stay in the hospital? Can you predict and prevent potential complications?

A killer and crippler
Despite the fact that cerebrovascular disease (CVD) ranks as one of mankind's greatest killers and cripplers, many of you have little preparation for caring for a patient who's been stricken by a stroke. Or you may have shied away from these patients because of CVD's high mortality rate. Yet, they're the ones who really need expert nursing care. Many doctors even say that the patient's prognosis depends largely on the quality of the care you give him.

On this page and the one opposite, you'll learn exactly what happens when a patient has a CVA — and what can cause it. Later on, I'll explain why stroke victims don't always have the same signs and symptoms — and why some recover better than others. But first, let's get back to the emergency department and the care you'll be giving to Sam Brand.

Making an assessment
As soon as you've determined that Mr. Brand has an open airway and is breathing adequately, you'll begin assessing the extent of his neurologic deficits. This initial assessment is important, because it serves as a baseline for future assessments. It gives others a way to measure any neurologic improvement he may show — or any deterioration. For this reason, document all your findings exactly. Besides providing a way to communicate, a well written assessment gives you a foundation on which to build an effective care plan.

In Chapter 2, you learned how to do a complete neurologic assessment. You'll follow these guidelines when you assess Mr. Brand's condition. But, because he may have suffered a CVA, you'll pay special attention to these areas:
• level of consciousness (LOC)
• motor and sensory functions
• cranial nerve function
• speech.

Testing Sam Brand's LOC
To test Mr. Brand's level of consciousness, you measure the minimal stimulus needed to elicit a response, as well as the

nature of that response. Mr. Brand responds quickly when you talk to him by nodding his head and attempting to talk. This is an appropriate and effective response, and you document it—giving *complete* details—on your assessment form.

Suppose Mr. Brand acted more lethargic? You might have to shake him to get a response and then find his response inappropriate. You'd document these details exactly, so the doctor will know precisely what occurred. How accurately you've documented specific details about your patient's level of consciousness is of *critical* importance to the doctor making the evaluation.

Why? Because changes in a patient's level of consciousness usually occur before changes in pupils or motor function. Thus, even subtle changes can herald a patient's improvement or deterioration. If a subsequent assessment reveals that Mr. Brand doesn't open his eyes when his name is called—or has to be shaken to be aroused—then his condition is deteriorating. You'd call the doctor immediately, reporting your findings in detail.

The patient's orientation to person, place, and time is something else you assess when you're observing his level of consciousness. In a patient like Mr. Brand, you'll probably find this difficult. He may know the correct answers to your questions but, because of his CVA, may be unable to express himself. *Nursing tip:* Solve this problem by asking the patient to nod yes or no as you give him a series of alternative answers to choose from.

Testing motor and sensory functions

Now, using the guidelines outlined in Chapter 2, assess Mr. Brand's motor and sensory functions. Simultaneously, test both his left side and right side, so you can compare the two. Not only will the doctor want to know if one side is weaker than the other, but he'll also need a report on the sensory responses in each area. Document your findings carefully. Remember, others will be using your notes later to determine possible changes in Mr. Brand's condition.

Nursing tip: Suppose you are examining a comatose patient. To tell which side of his body may be affected when he regains consciousness, test his response to painful stimuli. Consider little or no response to stimuli a positive indicator of paresis.

Hemorrhagic CVD
This problem may occur in all age groups. Rupture of a cerebral artery extravasates blood into or around the brain. As a result, blood supply to the area usually nourished is decreased, and the accumulation of blood may further compress the artery and damage surrounding cells. Hemorrhagic strokes are usually caused by coagulation defects, chronic hypertension, or by such vascular malformations as aneurysms, which are discussed in detail in Chapter 4.

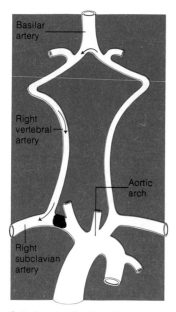

Subclavian steal syndrome
As you can see in the drawing above, an occlusion of the subclavian artery proximal to the origin of the vertebral artery will also block the vertebral artery's normal blood flow. To compensate for this occlusion, the patient's body diverts blood from the other vertebral artery and sends it *down* the ipsilateral vertebral artery instead, thereby "stealing" blood from the vertebrobasilar system.

When this occurs, the decreased supply of blood to the patient's brainstem and occipital lobe may produce symptoms of: decreased B.P. on affected arm; dizziness; light-headedness; blurred or double vision; facial numbness; loss of consciousness with exertion or when using the ipsilateral arm.

Some doctors may choose surgical treatment: usually, a bypass vein graft from the ipsilateral common carotid to the subclavian artery distal to the origin of the vertebral artery.

What about cranial nerve function?

Anytime a patient has a deficit in cranial nerve function, he'll have special problems that'll require both skill and ingenuity on your part to solve. If the deficit involves his optic nerves, which are part of the cranial nerves, he'll have a visual problem. A common visual problem that occurs in patients with cerebrovascular disease is field-cut—the loss of vision in a *portion* of each eye.

How can this happen? If you examine the picture opposite, you can see how the optic nerves cross at the optic chiasm in the brain. Because Mr. Brand's CVA affected his left optic tract, it resulted in loss of vision in the right half of each eye. This means he won't be able to see anything to his right unless he turns his head in that direction.

When Mr. Brand gets transferred to the ICU, he'll need a care plan designed to overcome the problems caused by this deficit. I'll tell you how to write this plan—and give him the care he needs—a little later in this chapter.

As you assess Mr. Brand in the emergency department, you also discover other cranial nerve deficits and document them. For example, when you ask him to smile and show his teeth, his mouth droops on the right side. This suggests facial nerve paresis, which means Mr. Brand will have trouble controlling secretions, taking medications, and eating and drinking with the right side of his mouth. To minimize his risk of aspirating his medication or food, place it on the back of his tongue or on the unimpaired side of his mouth. Then, turn his head toward the unimpaired side and give him a sip of water. *Important:* Always check the gag reflex in a patient with cerebrovascular disease. If it's not working properly, you can't feed him orally, because he may aspirate some of his food or liquid. You'll also have to suction his secretions regularly to prevent airway obstruction or pneumonia.

Covering all bases

Before you complete Mr. Brand's initial assessment—or the assessment of any patient with strokelike symptoms—find out if he has a stiff neck, a headache, or is sensitive to light. If he has any of these symptoms, the doctor will want to know about them. They all suggest meningeal irritation, which may be caused by intracranial bleeding or infection.

Nursing tip: Be alert for possible seizures in a patient with

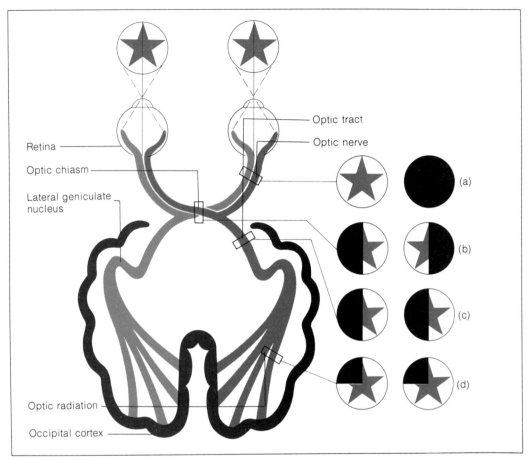

Retina

Optic chiasm

Lateral geniculate nucleus

Optic tract

Optic nerve

(a)

(b)

(c)

(d)

Optic radiation

Occipital cortex

Visual pathways

Patients with brain injuries or other intracranial lesions may suffer visual abnormalities. You'll find it easier to understand how the location of the lesion determines what it does to the patient's vision if you study the simplified illustration above.

As you can see, fibers emerge from the eyeball at the optic nerve. The neurons innervating the medial (nasal) half of each retina cross at the *optic chiasma;* those that supply the lateral (temporal) half continue back on the same side without crossing. From the optic tracts, impulses travel via the optic radiations through the temporal, parietal, and occipital lobes to the visual cortex in the occipital lobe.

This arrangement explains why:
• A lesion of the right optic nerve (a) creates total loss of vision in the right eye.
• A lesion of the optic chiasm (b) creates loss of vision in the lateral fields of both eyes.
• A lesion of the right optic tract (c) creates a loss of vision of the medial field of the right eye and the lateral field of the left eye.
• A partial lesion of the right optic radiation (d) may involve only a portion of the nerve fibers and create loss of vision in one-quarter of the visual field in each eye producing, for example, a homonymous *left* upper quadrantic defect.

Deficits of vision such as these are also referred to as *field-cuts.* You may need to remind your patient with a field-cut to turn his head frequently to compensate for his visual loss. In addition, he may have pain in the eyes, head, neck, shoulders, or back from the effort of doing this. Regular backrubs and medication may help.

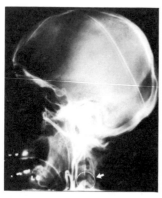

CVA assessment aids
Pictured above is an angiogram
indicating a thrombosis of the
left internal carotid artery.
 • *Angiography:* Helps determine the specific lesion causing
a CVA
 • *CAT scan:* To identify areas
of edema, hematomas, infarcts,
mass lesions, hydrocephalus
 • *Lumbar puncture:* To obtain
CSF; bloody or yellow-orange
color if stroke is hemorrhagic
 • *EEG:* To determine areas of
decreased cellular function and
potential for seizure activity
 • *Brain scan:* To show ischemic
area; may be negative for several days after stroke
 • *EKG:* To demonstrate heart
disease, if present; may be mild
ST-T wave changes early after
hemorrhagic stroke
 • *Cerebral blood flow studies*
(currently at only a few large
medical centers): To detect deficiencies in cerebral circulation
 • *Cerebral-evoked potential
testing:* To assess neurologic
changes after a stroke
 • *Doppler ultrasonography:* To
detect arteriovenous disease
impairing blood flow
 • *Laboratory studies:* To confirm diagnosis; studies include
urinalysis, coagulation studies,
CBC, serum electrolytes and
osmolality, serum glucose, triglycerides, creatinine, and BUN.

cerebrovascular disease. If one occurs, follow the instructions
in Chapter 9, and document your observations in detail.

Besides doing a neurologic assessment of your patient,
you must also assess his physical condition, paying particular
attention to his cardiovascular system. Naturally, you've already checked for an open airway and adequate respirations
before you started your neurologic assessment (especially important in lethargic patients). You've also completed a vital
signs check to rule out the possibility of other problems.

Important: Keep in mind that shock-type symptoms are
rarely caused by cerebrovascular disease. If your patient has
any, it means that he also has another problem; for example,
gastrointestinal bleeding, severe infection, or heart disease.

The final diagnosis

As important as the findings in your initial assessment are, the
doctor needs more information before he can diagnose Sam
Brand's problem. To get this information, he'll probably order
some or all of the tests listed on this page. (For a more complete description of these tests, and how to prepare your
patient for them, see the Appendices.)

After a thorough evaluation, the doctor decides that Mr.
Brand has suffered a CVA, involving the left middle cerebral
artery. You'll learn how it's possible to determine which of the
brain's arteries are involved further on in this chapter. But
first, imagine that your patient is transferred to the ICU, where
he'll receive care individualized to his needs.

If you were the nurse admitting Mr. Brand to the ICU, you'd
complete his assessment by interviewing him. You'd ask
about his past medical history, paying particular attention to
risk factors (see opposite page). You'd find out if he was taking
any medication, and you'd ask about his occupation, family,
and life-style.

From Mr. Brand and his ranch foreman, you learn that your
patient is a hard-driving perfectionist, who almost never re-
laxes. He smokes more than 2 packs of cigarettes a day, but
rarely drinks alcohol. He's been told by a doctor that he has
"high cholesterol," which he ignores on the grounds that it's
foolishness.

As you question Mr. Brand, you find out that he's experienced several episodes when his hand wouldn't "work right"
and his voice became slurred. These "spells" cleared after a

few minutes, and Mr. Brand attributed them to being tired.

However, you know that this suggests transient ischemic attacks (TIAs), which are really minor strokes or occlusions. In many cases, TIAs precede major occlusive strokes, so they mustn't be taken lightly. If a doctor had been called to evaluate these "spells," he may have been able to prevent Mr. Brand's major stroke.

Knowing what to expect

Before I get into the care you'll give Mr. Brand in the ICU, let me explain why stroke patients have different signs and symptoms. Why are some acutely ill and permanently disabled, while others recover quickly with no deficit? Five things determine the type and severity of symptoms:
- which cerebral artery was involved
- what portion of the brain was supplied by that artery and how it was affected
- how severe the damage was
- how large an area was damaged
- how well the brain compensated for the decreased blood supply. (See page 61 for more information about collateral circulation.)

As you recall, the doctor felt that Sam Brand had suffered a CVA that involved his left middle cerebral artery. His symptoms of right hemiparesis, aphasia, and visual field-cut (homonymous hemianopsia) correlate with those expected when there's damage to the brain area supplied by the left middle cerebral artery. Mr. Brand also lacks awareness of and has numbness on his affected side, although he'll probably have more weakness and numbness in his face and arm than his lower limbs.

Refer to page 21 to see the other arteries that supply the brain. I've already told you what symptoms to expect when the middle cerebral artery is involved. Now I'll list what symptoms occur in a patient with involvement of other arteries, so you can see how they vary. Document all symptoms in your assessment. It'll help the doctor locate the lesion, and help you plan the patient's care.
- *Carotid.* Ischemia to the brain area supplied by this artery can cause weakness, paralysis, numbness, sensory changes, and visual disturbances on the opposite side. Also, headache and altered level of consciousness. Bruits commonly occur.

Major risk factors in thrombotic CVD
- Atherosclerosis
- Heart disease
- Diabetes mellitus
- Hypertension
- High serum cholesterol or triglycerides
- Family history of stroke
- Obesity
- Sedentary life
- Oral contraceptives
- Cigarette smoking.
(Note the similarity between the risk factors for cerebrovascular disease and cardiovascular disease.)

Surgery

When the doctor chooses surgery for a CVA patient, he hopes to prevent further strokes, not treat the current stroke. Candidates are usually patients with transient ischemic attacks (TIAs), or with a completed stroke of mild-to-moderate degree. The most common surgical procedures are:

• *Carotid endarterectomy,* in which atherosclerotic plaques that might cause TIAs are removed from the inner arterial wall. The endarterectomy is usually performed at the bifurcation of the artery, where the plaques commonly occur.

Postop nursing tips:

— Because heparin is used during the procedure, be sure to observe carefully for postoperative hemorrhage.

— Check speech, level of consciousness, pupillary signs, motor functioning, and superior temporal artery pulse.

• *Microvascular bypass,* a relatively new procedure, may be used to improve intracranial circulation. Candidates may include patients with inaccessible carotid stenosis; vertebrobasilar stenosis or occlusion; or middle cerebral artery stenosis or occlusion. An extracranial vessel, such as the superficial temporal artery, is surgically anastomosed with an intracranial vessel, such as the middle cerebral artery. In this way, collateral circulation is created, bypassing the stenosis or occlusion.

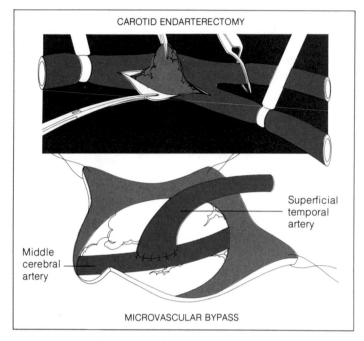

CAROTID ENDARTERECTOMY

Superficial temporal artery

Middle cerebral artery

MICROVASCULAR BYPASS

• *Vertibrobasilar.* Ischemia to the brain area supplied by this artery can cause one-sided weakness, numbness around mouth and lips, visual field-cut in one or both eyes (homonomous hemianopsia), double vision, poor coordination, clumsiness, slurred speech, difficulty swallowing, dizziness, vomiting, ataxia, and loss of memory.

• *Anterior cerebral artery.* Ischemia to the brain area supplied by this artery can cause weakness and numbness on the opposite side (especially in the lower extremities), incontinence, confusion, personality change, and the inability to perform certain purposeful movements (with loss of motor power, sensation, or coordination).

• *Posterior cerebral arteries.* Ischemia to the brain area supplied by these arteries can cause visual field-cuts in one or both eyes (homonomous hemianopsia), cortical blindness, sensory impairment, and dyslexia. In most cases, paralysis is absent.

How good a recovery your patient will make after a CVA is uncertain at first, because no one can tell exactly how many brain cells were killed by ischemia. As you know, when brain cells are deprived of oxygen, they die after a few minutes and no new cells develop to replace them. Of course, some cells may only be damaged, and these have potential for recovery. (Fortunately, collateral blood circulation sometimes makes it possible for other arteries to take over the work of the damaged artery and supply blood to the ischemic area before the cells die.)

Cell damage also results in edema with related symptoms, although these symptoms may disappear as the edema subsides.

Nursing tip: The quicker a stroke patient shows function return to the affected area, the better his chances are for a good recovery. No improvement after a few days is a poor sign.

Giving the CVA patient good care

As soon as the doctor's made his diagnosis, he'll decide what kind of treatment your patient will need for a good recovery. Since every case is different, the treatment ordered will vary too. In some cases he may recommend surgery, and in most he'll order some of the medications listed on page 63. But in all cases, he'll want the patient to receive top quality nursing care which, of course, is your responsibility.

Caring for a patient who's had a CVA can be extremely difficult. Why? Because his stroke has not only hurt him physically, but psychologically, as well. He may be partially or completely paralyzed — depending on the site and severity of his stroke — and he may be unable to speak. He may not even comprehend speech, and in many cases he'll have suffered personality changes.

Review the list of symptoms your patient may have on page 60. Is it any wonder that he's frustrated and depressed, and perhaps even emotionally unstable? I'll tell you how to deal with these behavior changes a little later in this chapter. But first, let's discuss the physical care your patient will need after he's admitted to the ICU.

The doctor will probably want you to do the following:

• Maintain adequate respiratory function. Make this your number one priority when you're caring for a stroke patient. His decreased level of consciousness, difficulty swallowing, or inability to control secretions are just a few of the things that can cause him to aspirate or develop other respiratory difficulties. To lessen this risk, change his position at least once every 2 hours, and encourage him to cough and deep-breathe.

Postop nursing tips:
To care for your CVA patient after he's had surgery:
— Check superficial temporal and carotid artery pulses.
— Check for infection or hemorrhage.
— Monitor blood pressure closely to maintain at optimum preop level. Deviations may lead to thrombosis or hemorrhage at the anastomotic site.
— Check neurologic signs for possible deficits. They may indicate an ischemic attack.
— Anticipate aspirin therapy for 4 to 6 weeks to prevent clumping of platelets at the anastomotic site.
— Position the patient so he doesn't lie on the operative side. Doing so may help prevent occlusion.

Danger signals
Any of these conditions in CVA patients may indicate a serious, perhaps life-threatening situation:
• Deteriorating level of consciousness
• Respiratory changes with blood-gas deterioration
• Blood pressure spikes
• Onset, recurrence, worsening of motor deficits
• Onset, recurrence, worsening of vision difficulties
• Onset, recurrence, worsening of speech problems.

Suction secretions to prevent pneumonia — the most common cause of death in CVA patients — and airway obstruction. Keep lethargic patients in a head-down, lateral position to allow secretions to drain naturally. But remember to alternate the side he's lying on at least once every 2 hours. Watch for signs of pulmonary embolus, another dangerous complication.

In most cases, a stroke patient will have had his blood-gas levels measured on admission. But if he's comatose, he'll need them measured frequently. *Important:* Anytime you see that a patient's PCO_2 level is rising or that his PO_2 level is falling, call the doctor immediately. He may order endotracheal intubation or possibly even a tracheotomy.

• Watch for signs of increased intracranial pressure. This may develop secondary to intracranial hemorrhage or the edema associated with a severe stroke. To learn how to assess and deal with this problem, see the discussion of increased intracranial pressure in Chapter 5.

• Maintain fluid and electrolyte balance. For a short time at least, your stroke patient will receive I.V. fluids to keep a vein open in case he needs medication. How much fluid he'll receive depends on his electrolyte and osmolality status. When you're caring for a stroke patient, never administer a large amount of fluid in a short time. Carefully monitor his serum electrolyte values, and keep accurate intake and output records.

• Check blood pressure frequently. Blood pressure elevations after a stroke are common, but usually return to normal after the patient's been hospitalized for 24 hours. However, if his diastolic blood pressure stays over 100 mm Hg, call the doctor. He may order an antihypertensive drug. Was your patient's stroke caused by hemorrhage? A sudden blood pressure spike may be a warning of an impending rebleed. Notify the doctor at once.

• Continue neurologic assessment. In the first few days after a CVA, changes can occur quite suddenly, so make neurologic checks hourly. Record your findings accurately on a neurologic flow sheet, and immediately report any decline in function to the doctor.

• Monitor urinary output. Since stroke patients are particularly prone to urinary infections, the doctor will want to avoid ordering a Foley catheter for conscious patients. Do all you can to keep your patient from requiring catheterization.

Don't wait for him to ask for the urinal. Offer it every 2 hours and after he's had liquids. Make sure he understands what you mean. Remember, he may have trouble comprehending speech. If you suspect this may be true, use an illustrated card to convey the idea.

• Ensure adequate nutrition. Although comatose and lethargic patients may be fed by nasogastric tube, many stroke patients can receive oral feedings. Some patients may even be able to feed themselves, depending on the degree of motor damage sustained.

In any case always make sure your patient's gag reflex is working before you give him an oral feeding. If one side of his face is paralyzed, remember that — even with a soft diet — he'll have a lot of trouble eating and drinking because that side of his mouth is numb. Food and liquids may drip from the corner of his mouth without him realizing it. This can be very distressing to a patient and his family, so be patient and reassuring. *Nursing tip:* The patient who wears dentures may complain that they continually come loose on his affected side, adding to his embarrassment. Tell him that this is because he no longer chews as much on that side and help remedy the situation with denture adhesive.

At first, your patient may find it easier to manage semisolid foods, because he can control them better than liquids in his mouth. He may also have less difficulty eating if he lies on his side, with his unaffected side down.

Suppose your patient has a visual field-cut because of his stroke. Be sure to place his food tray and basin on his unaffected side, so he can see it easily. Document the way to arrange things on his care plan so they'll stay the same on every shift.

• Manage gastrointestinal problems, preventing them when possible. Watch for possible vomiting in the first few days after a CVA, and keep your patient positioned on his side with his head down so he doesn't aspirate his vomitus. Keep in mind he might be constipated, in which case the doctor will probably order stool softeners. Check his stools for bleeding, because stroke patients are prone to stress ulcers.

• Provide proper mouth care. Oral hygiene is important, particularly for the unconscious patient or one with facial nerve paresis or paralysis. Because food can easily accumulate on the affected side, clean and irrigate your patient's

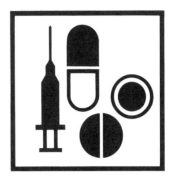

Medications for CVA patients
Medications that may be routinely given to patients with CVA are:

• *Anticonvulsants:* Dilantin or phenobarbital, to prevent or treat seizures

• *Antihypertensives:* When diastolic pressure's greater than 110 mm Hg or after hypertensive strokes

• *Steroids:* Treatment of associated cerebral edema

• *Stool softeners*

• *Analgesics:* Codeine for severe headache after hemorrhagic stroke (aspirin may be contraindicated for hemorrhagic patients because it can prolong bleeding time)

• *Vasodilators for occlusive CVA*

• *Anticoagulants or aspirin:* To prevent or treat pulmonary emboli and deep vein thrombosis. (These drugs contraindicated if CVA's cause is hemorrhage.)

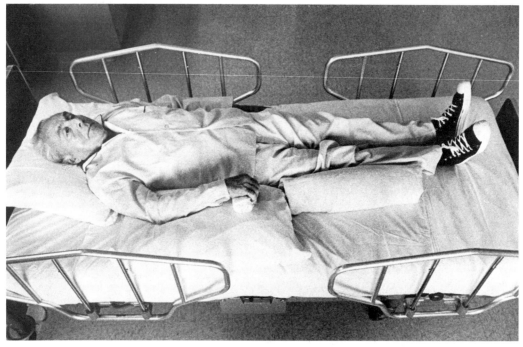

Rehabilitation

For the patient who's suffered a CVA, rehabilitation begins as soon as you begin caring for him. This means that during the acute phase of your patient's illness, you must take *preventive* measures to avoid severe, perhaps irreversible complications. Not doing so will prolong your patient's dependency on others.

The most likely complications to occur are *contractures* and *skin breakdown*. To learn how to prevent them, read these pages and study the accompanying illustrations.

Positioning

Follow these positioning guidelines to prevent contractures, pressure sores, and respiratory problems in your patient. Doing so will add to his comfort and safety.

• *Prone and semiprone:* Either of these positions is helpful if your patient with a CVA develops lung congestion, because they promote bronchial drainage.

• *Supine:* Use this position when patient's alert. Because skin and contracture problems are more likely to occur with this position, be sure to take these precautions.

— Head: Place a *small* pillow under the patient's head for support. Using a bulky pillow (or more than one) can force his head downward, causing a contracture. *It may even interfere with his breathing.*

— Upper extremities: Look at the patient's arm in the above photo. Note that the affected elbow is pointed away from the trunk and is slightly bent. The lower arm and the hand extend alongside the trunk about 12" away. Change this arm position at intervals by extending the elbow. To prevent edema, use a pillow to elevate the arm. Place a small rolled object in the patient's paralyzed hand to help prevent clenched hand deformity. You may remove this periodically and extend the fingers.

— Trunk: Align the body with the spine straight, shoulders level with hips.

— Lower extremities: Make sure your patient's legs are straight. You may place a trochanter roll along the outside of his affected thigh. This prevents the hip from rolling outward (external rotation). You may make the trochanter roll from a bath blanket, pillow, or covered foam rubber. Don't use sandbags, which may lead to serious skin-breakdown problems.

Don't routinely put pillows under the patient's knees or keep the knee gatch of his bed elevated. This can produce knee contractures and increase hip contracture. Remember, gravity will pull your patient's paralyzed

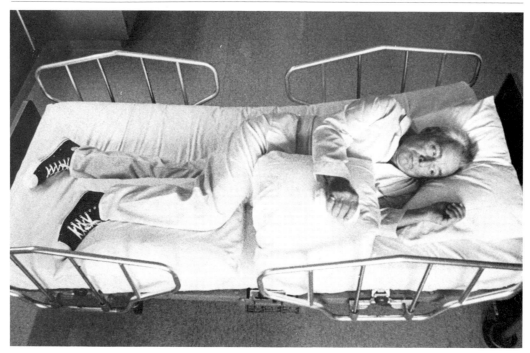

foot into a footdrop position, shortening his calf muscles and heel cords. To prevent this, try one of the following precautions:

Use a *footboard* to support his feet at a 90° angle. It should be about 2 inches higher than the toes. Place the feet against it with toes pointed toward the ceiling. Allow enough space between the edge of the mattress and the footboard to avoid undue pressure on the heels. *Note:* You may have difficulty keeping the feet against the board.

Other alternatives:

Use *Spenco boots* to keep the feet aligned at a 90° angle and to prevent pressure on the heels and lateral maleoli.

Use *high-top tennis sneakers* to maintain dorsiflexion (upward flexion). Some feel they keep the feet in a more normal anatomical position. *Be sure to remove them from time to time to inspect for skin breakdown.*

Use *splints* on your patient's affected extremities to maintain proper alignment. For nursing care, see page 115.

• *Side-lying position:* Particularly good for preventing contractures and respiratory problems. *Use this position if your patient's unconscious.* If you position him so that he's lying on his affected side, make sure he doesn't remain in this position for too long.

— Head: You may use a pillow under the head to promote comfort and maintain proper alignment.

— Trunk: Keep the spine straight. Place a pillow at your patient's back for support, although it's not essential if he's positioned properly.

— Upper extremities: Bring the uppermost arm forward in front of the patient. Bend his elbow slightly, but keep his wrist extended. Support his arm on a pillow and bring the bottom arm

up alongside the face with palm up. You may place a small roll in the affected hand.

— Lower extremities: Flex the uppermost leg and bring it forward. Support it on pillows to prevent internal rotation (rolling forward) of the hip. Keep the lower leg extended straight and level with the spine. To avoid possible pressure sores, make sure your patient's top leg doesn't rest on his lower leg. Take precautions to prevent footdrop.

Your patient can develop contractures like those illustrated on page 66 unless you take great care to prevent them. As you know, unequal strength in opposing sets of muscles fosters contractures. The arm adducts (held close to the trunk); the shoulder internally rotates with flexion of the forearm, wrists, and fingers (clawlike hand). Note the externally rotated hip, flexed knee, and development of

**Contractures:
An avoidable
complication**

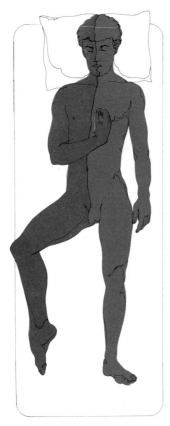

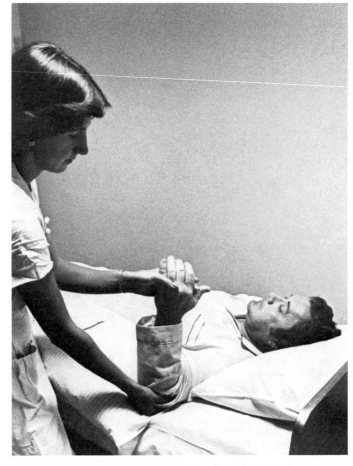

footdrop. *Always position to counteract these tendencies.*

If your patient's unconscious or has bilateral paralysis, you can still follow these position guidelines. Just apply the suggestions for one side of the body to both sides.

Range-of-motion exercises
To increase your patient's circulation, maintain his joint mobility, and prevent contractures, follow these exercise guidelines:
1. Begin your patient's exercise program *as soon as he's admitted,* unless his doctor says otherwise.
2. Find out if your patient has any existing health problems that might affect his joint motion and thwart your goals for him — for example, arthritis.
3. Consult with the doctor and physical therapist to set up an individualized exercise program for your patient.
4. If your patient's unconscious, perform passive exercises on each extremity.
5. When he's regained consciousness, perform passive exercises on affected extremities; encourage active exercises of nonaffected extremities.
6. Determine *your patient's* full range of motion. To do this, note the point at which any movement meets with resistance or causes pain. Never use force to exceed these limits. Always stop whenever the patient shows signs of pain.
7. Always perform exercise motions gently, slowly and rhythmically.
8. Make sure your patient's body is aligned properly while he's exercising.
9. Repeat each passive exercise three times during an exercise

Rehabilitation

period, unless instructed otherwise.

10. Carry out the exercise program (at least twice) daily. Consider the patient's daily activities and preferences when planning his schedule.

11. Modify your initial program, as needed. For example, if you notice your patient's arm beginning to adduct, emphasize shoulder abduction and external rotation.

12. Explain your patient's exercise program in detail in his nursing care plan.

13. If your patient develops a deformity or *shows further losses of mobility,* notify the doctor.

Skin care

Follow these skin-care guidelines to increase circulation and prevent skin breakdown:

• *Positioning:* At first, set a 2-hour limit for each position. Then make adjustments based on your observations. When you change your patient's position, check for skin redness where he's been resting. Temporary redness is normal in areas subjected to pressure. If redness persists after 30 minutes, decrease the time he spends in that position. If redness doesn't disappear shortly or if skin is broken, avoid all pressure on this site, and eliminate the position entirely for a time.

If the patient's skin shows no signs of redness after a position change, you may increase the time he spends in that position. However, do so gradually, ½ hour at a time, to a maximum of 4 hours in any position.

Be sure to document all changes on his nursing care plan.

• *Massage:* After a position change, stimulate circulation by carefully massaging those areas where there's been pressure. The chart above shows which areas are most apt to break down. They'll need extra attention.

When massaging, use firm —

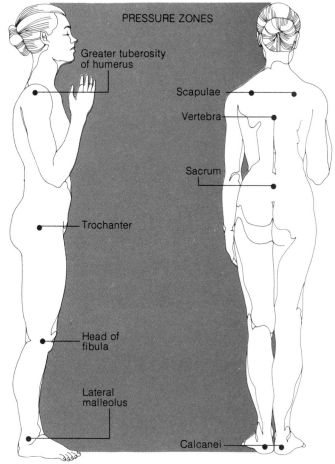

PRESSURE ZONES

Greater tuberosity of humerus

Scapulae

Vertebra

Sacrum

Trochanter

Head of fibula

Lateral malleolus

Calcanei

but not hard — pressure. Make circular movements over the entire area, repeating the process 5 to 6 times.

Caution: If you notice signs of incipient breakdown, *massage around, but not over the area.*

— Special protection aids such as sheepskins, egg-crate pads, and water beds help prevent skin breakdown. Check to see which are available and obtain them. Remember, however, that appliances, special dressings, and lotions are no substitute for a positioning and massage plan.

— If your patient has special positioning aids such as tennis sneakers or splints, remove them periodically to inspect and massage the site.

Looking to the future

Following an effective care plan like this one can save your patient from skin breakdown and contractures. By preventing such complications, you'll be helping him towards an earlier recovery. Thanks to your care, he'll be able to participate more actively in a later and more demanding rehabilitative program.

mouth after he eats to remove food particles. To do this properly, first remove his dentures (if he has any), then turn him so that his affected side is uppermost. Brush your patient's teeth with a child's toothbrush. Now fill a large syringe with 3 parts mouthwash and 1 part hydrogen peroxide, and put a 2″ plastic I.V. catheter on the end for a soft, flexible irrigating tip. Then get someone to suction his mouth while you irrigate it with the peroxide-mouthwash solution.

• Give eye care. If your patient's corneal reflexes aren't working properly, he'll need special eye care to prevent corneal abrasion. To provide this, moisten cotton balls with normal saline solution and use them to remove secretions from his eyes every 4 hours. The doctor may also order special lubricating eye drops. Keep the affected eye taped closed with Steri-Strips placed horizontally. Caution: Some doctors feel it's dangerous to use a patch or eye shield because the patient's eye might open underneath, without your knowing it.

• Prevent skin breakdown and other complications of immobility. Because your stroke patient will probably be hospitalized for some time, he'll need special attention in these areas if he's to make a good recovery. To give him the kind of quality care he needs, see the guidelines on rehabilitation on pages 64 through 67.

Understanding your patient's behavior

As I said earlier, the brain damage caused by your patient's stroke may not only affect him physically, but mentally. Depending on the site of the lesion, he may have personality changes caused by ischemia. These changes will affect his behavior and may cause many difficult problems.

For example, he'll probably be depressed. (This would be understandable even without brain damage, considering that he no longer can care for himself completely and must be dependent on others.) As his depression deepens, he may withdraw and lose interest in getting better. He may even regress to emotional outbursts and childlike behavior.

Help your patient avoid or overcome long depressions by including him in his own care from the very start. In other words, let him make some decisions when possible. Treat and think of him as an adult human being with fears and frustrations, rather than just another CVA patient. Take time to let him and his family know that you care about their feelings and

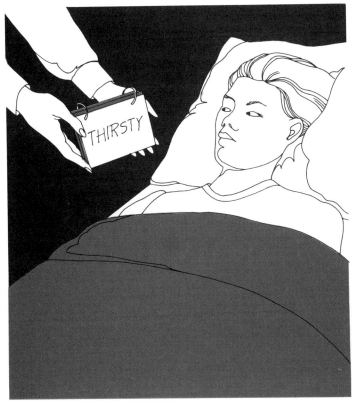

Aphasia

When a patient's brain becomes damaged from a CVA, he may suffer aphasia, which is a loss of power to express or comprehend language. Depending on where the lesion is, aphasia can be of the *expressive* type, in which the patient has difficulty expressing what he thinks; or the *receptive* type, in which he has trouble understanding what people are telling him.

For example, the patient with expressive aphasia has trouble naming objects and using the correct words to express himself. What's more, he may also have difficulty expressing himself in writing. The patient with receptive aphasia will have trouble reading, following even simple instructions, and recognizing people and things. As a result, his verbal responses may not always be appropriate. Sometimes patients will have a combination of these two types.

Many patients with aphasia recover some of their ability to speak and comprehend during the first several months after a CVA. But even if such spontaneous recovery is very good, progress can be improved if a speech therapist works with the patient. Speech therapy should begin as soon as the patient is physically able. The speech therapist can also give tips to you and the patient's family so you can better communicate with him, as well as suggestions on how to help him.

Ten tips on communicating with the aphasic patient

1. Talk to your patient as an adult; aphasia doesn't mean he has lost his intelligence.
2. Speak slowly and use simple, short sentences along with gestures, when possible.
3. Don't shout; hearing loss is not part of aphasia and shouting will not help the patient understand.
4. Speak to the patient frequently; don't neglect him because he doesn't understand what you say or has trouble communicating — this approach may cause him to feel isolated and he may withdraw into silence.
5. Be honest with your patient; don't pretend you understand if you don't. He may be trying to tell you something important.
6. Remember, your patient may be experiencing extreme frustration as he attempts and fails to perform tasks that were previously routine. Anticipate displays of emotion as he tries to cope with incapacity, and offer him your reassurance as these feelings surface.
7. Avoid the tendency to talk for the patient or frequently supply him with words; have patience with his efforts, slow as they may be.
8. Check whether the patient has auditory comprehension by asking him a question that requires a "no" answer; he's more likely to answer "yes" to all questions. For example, "Did you have soup for breakfast this morning?"
9. Use a set of cards with words such as "bedpan," "thirsty," or "hurt," to help the patient communicate needs and reduce frustration. Encourage him to communicate by writing, if he's able. (Don't use these approaches alone, without efforts to communicate verbally.)
10. Avoid tiring the patient; aphasia gets worse with fatigue or emotional upset.

welfare, and are willing to help them through a difficult time.

Don't reinforce his negative feelings about his altered body image by referring to affected areas as "your bad side" or "your crippled leg." Use only the words "right" and "left," because these are nonjudgmental.

Does your patient seem disoriented to time and place? Encourage his family to bring him a small clock, cheerful calendar, and some family pictures. Then make a point to talk about these things when you enter his room.

Use your own imagination and ingenuity to help your patient overcome his difficulties. And above all, be reassuring and positive when you speak to him and his family. Don't let conversations center on how things were before his CVA. Instead, keep everyone looking at the future, anticipating and finding satisfaction in each improvement.

Meeting the challenge

Does this sound challenging? It is. But you can meet this challenge successfully if you put your mind to it. Prepare your patient for his return home by carefully instructing him and his family. To help you do this, provide the family with the special booklets on strokes prepared by the American Heart Association. Then go over some of the special problems they'll face so they can make the necessary adjustments.

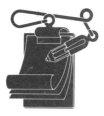

Remember these important points when caring for a patient who's suffered a CVA:

1. Be sure to accurately document specific details about your patient's level of consciousness. Subtle changes in consciousness level may provide the first indication of an improvement or deterioration in his condition.

2. Assess your patient for signs of a stiff neck, headache, or abnormal sensitivity to light. Any of these signs may indicate meningeal irritation, which can result from intracranial bleeding or infection.

3. Be aware that surgery for a CVA patient is aimed at preventing further strokes, not treating the current stroke.

4. Remember that the quicker a stroke patient shows function return to an affected area, the better his chances are for a good recovery. No improvement after a few days is a poor sign.

5. Prevent complications by following the proper guidelines for positioning, skin care, and range-of-motion exercises.

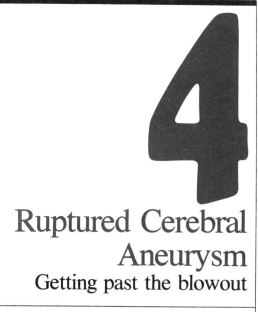

Ruptured Cerebral Aneurysm
Getting past the blowout

BY KATHLEEN A. BREUNIG, RN, BSN

YOU CAN SEE THAT Mr. Ott is greatly distressed. And it's understandable, because his 50-year-old wife Mabel has just been admitted to the hospital after suffering a ruptured cerebral aneurysm.

"It happened real suddenly," he whispers. "She just moaned, grabbed her head, and passed out...." When you ask him if she had any symptoms prior to this, he answers, "No, she was feeling fine."

Since you've already read the initial report on Mrs. Ott, you know that she's lethargic, but arousable. She responds to her name by opening her eyes, and her pupils are equal and react to light. She has mild nuchal rigidity, with weakness in her left arm, leg, and left lower facial muscles. A lumbar puncture done in the E.D. revealed grossly bloody cerebrospinal fluid with elevated pressure.

The doctor orders that Mrs. Ott be placed on bedrest with subarachnoid precautions. Do you know what he means? Specifically, how do you care for a patient with a subarachnoid hemorrhage? What observations should you make? What can you do to help minimize the risk of increased intracranial pressure?

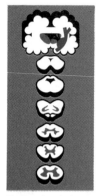

Pathophysiology
An aneurysm is a localized dilatation of an artery resulting from a weakness in the arterial wall. The weakness may be congenital, the effect of a degenerative process, or a combination of both. The defect may not appear until middle life, when hypertension and arteriosclerosis increase the turbulence and irregularity of blood flow. Then the weakened vessel wall balloons from the increasing pressure; its layers fray; its dome grows thin; and it may rupture at any time.

Among intracranial aneurysms, the most common is the saccular or berry type; it generally occurs at bifurcations of the arteries comprising the circle of Willis (see opposite page). A rupture here almost invariably results in a subarachnoid hemorrhage, in which extravasated blood reaches the subarachnoid space normally occupied by CSF.

Some ruptures, however, may produce intracerebral hemorrhages, bleeding into the brain tissues, with subsequent clot formation. A massive cerebral hemorrhage might involve less than 50 ml of blood, but the sharp increase in ICP and destruction of brain tissue can be fatal.

What early danger signs warn you of rebleeding, vasospasm, and tentorial herniation?

I'm going to discuss these in this chapter, so you'll know what to do for a patient like Mrs. Ott. I'll also explain which diagnostic procedures she'll undergo, what drugs she'll receive, and how surgery may help her.

When an aneurysm ruptures
Occasionally, a patient may have some headaches and episodes of drooping eyelid a few days before suffering a ruptured aneurysm. But, usually, subarachnoid hemorrhage gives little or no warning. Classically, its onset is explosive, with a sudden, severe headache, nausea and vomiting, and some degree of loss of consciousness. Depending on the severity of bleeding, the patient's level of consciousness can range from almost no change to deep coma (see page 34).

What happens when a cerebral aneurysm ruptures? As the blood accumulates in the subarachnoid space, meningeal irritation creates (and is revealed by) stiffness in the neck, pain down the back and into the legs, temperature elevation, restlessness, and irritability. Besides this, a patient may also be drowsy or confused, have visual disturbances, and possibly suffer a seizure.

Where the aneurysm is located also affects the symptoms a patient will have. Let's suppose, for example, the aneurysm bleeds into the brain's tissue. This may cause hemiparesis, visual disturbances, and dysphasia. If it enlarges or ruptures near the internal carotid artery, it may produce a third-nerve palsy by compression. This may cause double vision, because the patient can't use his affected eye muscles to look up, down, or medially. With third-nerve involvement, the patient may also have drooping eyelid (ptosis) and pupil dilation.

Confirming the diagnosis
As you already know, Mrs. Ott had a lumbar puncture, which showed bloody cerebrospinal fluid and increased pressure. This confirmed the doctor's diagnosis of subarachnoid hemorrhage, although it didn't necessarily indicate the presence of an aneurysm.

Mrs. Ott will require further diagnostic tests; for example, skull X-rays, computerized axial tomogram (CAT scan), and a cerebral angiogram. Of these, the cerebral angiogram is the

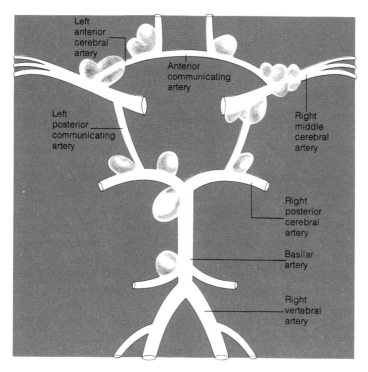

Left anterior cerebral artery

Anterior communicating artery

Left posterior communicating artery

Right middle cerebral artery

Right posterior cerebral artery

Basilar artery

Right vertebral artery

Locating cerebral aneurysms
This illustration, which includes the circle of Willis, shows the most common sites of cerebral aneurysms.

prime study done to confirm cerebral aneurysm, because it can usually locate a suspected aneurysm or even vasospasm. The CAT scan may also reveal a large aneurysm, but is primarily used to rule out other lesions that may cause subarachnoid hemorrhage. Skull X-rays may show calcification in the walls of a large aneurysm, or — rarely — some bone erosion of the skull. Other laboratory tests the doctor may order include CBC, urinalysis, coagulation studies, serum osmolality, and serum electrolyte and glucose levels.

Chances are, the doctor will also want the patient's blood-gas measurements checked. When you do this, be alert for high PCO_2 levels, which may cause increased intracranial pressure due to the vasodilating effect of the carbon dioxide. Watch also for low PO_2 levels, which indicate poor tissue perfusion.

Three major threats
The cerebral aneurysm patient faces three major threats: the initial bleed; rebleeding from the same site; and vasospasm.

Grading aneurysms
The severity of symptoms from ruptured cerebral aneurysm varies with the size and profuseness of the bleed. Here are descriptive categories:
• Grade I — mild bleed; alert, minimal headache, slight nuchal rigidity, no neurologic deficit
• Grade II — mild bleed; alert; mild-to-severe headache; nuchal rigidity; minimal neurologic deficit as a third nerve palsy
• Grade III — moderate bleed; drowsy or confused; nuchal rigidity; may have mild focal deficit
• Grade IV — moderate or severe bleed; stuporous; nuchal rigidity; may have mild-to-severe hemiparesis
• Grade V — severe bleed; in deep coma; decerebrate movements; possibly moribund.

The initial bleed. When Mrs. Ott's aneurysm ruptured and she first lost consciousness, the forceful release of arterial blood in the subarachnoid space was in itself quite damaging to the central nervous system. Then as the blood escaped into the brain tissue, it could form a life-threatening clot. The increased intracranial pressure might also cause brain tissue to shift downward, displacing brain stem structures and possibly cutting off the blood supply supporting vital functions (see Chapter 5).

Rebleeding. After the initial bleeding episode, a patient like Mrs. Ott risks bleeding again. After the leakage of 10 to 20 ml of blood, bleeding usually stops and a clot seals over the rupture, reinforcing the aneurysm for 7 to 10 days. However, around the 7th day, the clot begins to undergo the natural lytic process, and the chances of rebleeding from the same site rise.

If the patient's aneurysm rebleeds, she's faced with the same dangers she faces during the initial bleed. *Caution:* Keep in mind that *anything* that elevates blood pressure anytime after the first episode can cause rebleeding. Monitor your patient closely, and follow the precautions I'll explain later in this chapter.

Vasospasm. When vasospasm occurs in a patient, it indicates the constriction of intracranial blood vessels from smooth-muscle contraction. Vasospasm's cause is unknown, but it usually occurs in the vessel adjacent to the ruptured aneurysm. Depending on its intensity, it may spread through the major vessels at the base of the brain. This results in ischemia and possible infarction of involved areas, which will alter the functions controlled by those areas.

Caution: Watch for the symptoms of vasospasm shortly after the patient's initial bleed and also after surgical repair of the aneurysm. Call the doctor immediately if your patient develops hemiparesis, visual disturbances, seizures, or decreasing level of consciousness.

Two other life-threatening problems that commonly can occur in a patient with a ruptured cerebral aneurysm are these: pulmonary embolism and acute hydrocephalus. (For more information on your role dealing with acute hydrocephalus, read the discussion on page 137.)

Mrs. Ott had a clip applied to her aneurysm. But before she did, she was treated with complete bedrest and various drugs to control intracranial pressure. (For complete details on these

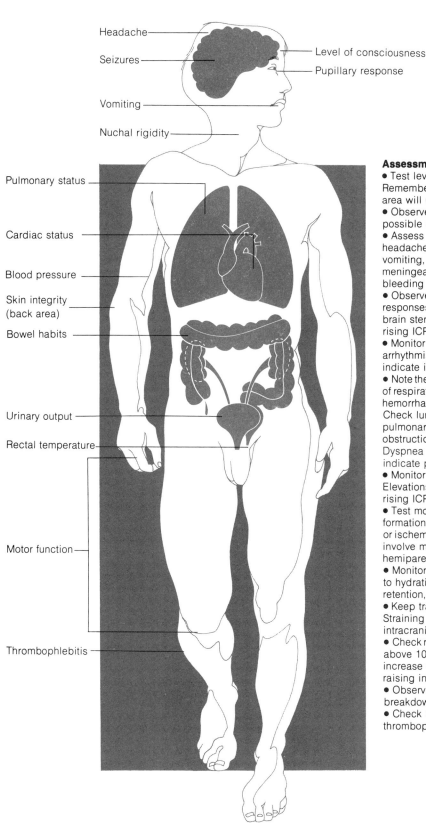

Headache

Seizures

Vomiting

Nuchal rigidity

Level of consciousness

Pupillary response

Pulmonary status

Cardiac status

Blood pressure

Skin integrity
(back area)

Bowel habits

Urinary output

Rectal temperature

Motor function

Thrombophlebitis

Assessment
● Test level of consciousness.
Remember, deterioration in this
area will usually occur *first*.
● Observe for seizures indicating
possible cerebral lesion.
● Assess carefully symptoms of
headache, nuchal rigidity, and
vomiting, which can indicate
meningeal irritation from
bleeding or infection.
● Observe the pupillary
responses. Changes may suggest
brain stem involvement from
rising ICP.
● Monitor EKG pattern for
arrhythmias. Bradycardia may
indicate increased ICP.
● Note the rate, depth, and pattern
of respirations. Increase in ICP or
hemorrhage may change them.
Check lung sounds for signs of
pulmonary complications. Airway
obstruction can raise ICP.
Dyspnea and chest pain can
indicate pulmonary embolus.
● Monitor B.P. for fluctuations.
Elevations in B.P. can reflect
rising ICP, rebleeding.
● Test motor function. The
formation of an intracerebral clot
or ischemia from vasospasm may
involve motor fibers and cause
hemiparesis.
● Monitor urinary output for clues
to hydration status as well as
retention, infection.
● Keep track of bowel habits.
Straining can increase
intracranial pressure.
● Check rectal temperature. A rise
above 101.5° F. (38.6° C.) will
increase cerebral blood flow,
raising intracranial pressure.
● Observe skin for evidence of
breakdown.
● Check legs for symptoms of
thrombophlebitis.

Danger signals
Any of these conditions in patients with cerebral aneurysm may indicate a serious, perhaps life-threatening, situation:
• Decrease in level of consciousness
• Unilateral enlarged pupil
• Onset of hemiparesis or worsening of a previous motor deficit
• Elevation in blood pressure
• Slowing pulse rate
• Sudden new headache or worsening headache
• Renewed or increased nuchal rigidity
• Persistent or renewed episode of vomiting.

drugs used to treat patients with a ruptured cerebral aneurysm or other conditions causing increased intracranial pressure, see Chapters 3 and 5.)

Knowing what nursing measures to take
Now let's talk about the specific care you'll be giving a patient like Mrs. Ott when she comes to your unit. In her case, the results of her cerebral angiography reveal an aneurysm on the right middle cerebral artery — with a resultant intracerebral clot. Because she's also developed a severe vasospasm of the entire right carotid system, her doctor delays surgical repair of her aneurysm until the vasospasm can be resolved. Until then, Mrs. Ott is given aminocaproic acid (Amicar) I.V. to delay clot lysis and hopefully prevent rebleeding (see opposite page).

What measures must you take to control Mrs. Ott's intracranial pressure and prevent further complications from occurring until she's ready for surgery. For most patients who've suffered a cerebral aneurysm, the doctor will order the following:

• *Establish and maintain an open airway.* As you already know, brain tissue, in particular, is very susceptible to oxygen deficit, and the least hypoxia from inadequate respiratory exchange will compound the existing injury by increasing intracranial pressure. In some cases, the doctor may order the patient intubated. If this happens, do nasotracheal suctioning as needed to keep the patient's lungs free of secretions — thus permitting proper gas exchange. Continue to monitor his blood-gas measurements regularly. Don't permit smoking in the patient's room, under any circumstances.

• *Monitor the patient's neurological status and record your findings.* Using the guidelines on page 75 and your baseline assessment as a reference point, monitor your patient's neurologic status at least hourly in the initial posthemorrhage period. Watch for any changes in his condition (see the danger signs listed on this page). These can indicate an enlarging aneurysm, rebleeding, an intracranial clot, vasospasm, or other complications.

• *Bedrest (with limited activity).* This is essential, because stress and activity elevate arterial blood pressure, which, in turn, can potentiate rebleeding from the aneurysm.

Be sure your patient has a darkened, quiet environment and try to anticipate all of his physiologic needs. To facilitate ve-

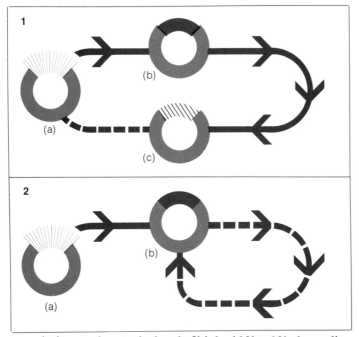

Amicar (aminocaproic acid)
Fig. 1. a) Ruptured aneurysm results in bleeding. b) Bleeding stops. Clot seals the rupture, reinforcing aneurysm. c) In 7 to 10 days, fibrinolysis normally occurs, dissolving the clot and creating the danger of rebleed. Fig. 2: a) Ruptured aneurysm results in bleeding. b) Bleeding stops. Clot seals the rupture, reinforcing aneurysm. Some doctors use Amicar during acute period to maintain this seal. An antifibrinolytic agent, Amicar delays clot dissolution and may forestall a potential rebleed.
• If the patient is receiving the drug I.V., *avoid infusing too rapidly.* If you don't, the result may be bradycardia, hypotension, or arrhythmias.
Tip: Use an I.V. infusion pump to control rate of administration.
• Observe patients receiving Amicar for these possible side effects: nausea, cramps, diarrhea, dizziness, tinnitus, headache, skin rash.
• Remember, antifibrinolytic activity may increase risk of thrombophlebitis and pulmonary embolus.

nous drainage, elevate the head of his bed 20° to 30°, depending on the doctor's orders.

Encourage your patient to rest and sleep as much as possible. The doctor may order a sedative such as phenobarbital. It also acts as an anticonvulsant. In cases where the patient's headache is severe, the doctor may also order an analgesic, such as codeine.

Caution: If you think oversedation is masking the patient's true level of consciousness, report this to the doctor, so he can reduce the medication.

Explain to your patient why his activities are restricted. Make sure he understands what you've told him and enlist his family's cooperation. Limit the number of visitors the patient has and take care that they don't upset him.

Keep in mind that your patient may be confused or behave inappropriately because of neurologic deficits caused by his ruptured aneurysm. Inform his family of this possibility. Employ the usual safety measures to prevent the patient from falling; for example, raised side rails, and lowered bed.

Caution: Don't use restraints, unless absolutely necessary, because they may further agitate the patient. This, in turn,

Hazards for aneurysm patients
Pulmonary emboli threaten any immobilized patient, but especially the patient with a ruptured cerebral aneurysm. He'll be particularly susceptible if he's getting an antifibrinolytic drug like aminocaproic acid (Amicar) to delay clot lysis. Because the patient's activity is restricted, fit him with elastic stockings or Ace bandages immediately after admission and use them until activity is resumed.

Should emboli occur despite all precautions, they usually bring chest pains, shortness of breath, dusky color, low PO$_2$ levels, tachycardia, fever, and a change in the patient's sensorium. Watch for any of these — changes may be subtle — and report them at once.

Treatment of emboli is usually through anticoagulant therapy, which is particularly dangerous for the aneurysm patient because it increases the chances of rebleeding at the aneurysm site. Be sure to:
● Observe for bleeding tendencies by checking all stool, emesis, and sputum for blood.
● Report at once any change in neurologic status.
● Maintain pulmonary hygiene and monitor arterial blood gas measurements to ensure adequate oxygenation.

Hydrocephalus, an engorgement of cerebrospinal fluid (CSF) in the cerebral ventricles, may follow a subarachnoid hemorrhage.

For a fuller discussion of hydrocephalus, see page 137.

may elevate his blood pressure and increase intracranial pressure.

Despite restrictions, the patient with a cerebral aneurysm must have some activity to prevent skin breakdown and minimize the risk of pulmonary complications. Make sure he turns — or is turned — every 2 hours, but ensure that all movements are gentle and unhurried. *Important:* Encourage your patient to breathe deeply, but remind him that coughing or sneezing may be dangerous.

If the doctor permits, your patient can perform active range-of-motion exercises every 2 hours. However, for some patients who are partly paralyzed, active exercises are impossible. In these cases, exercise the affected leg more than once every 2 hours to prevent thrombus formation. *Nursing tip:* Encourage all patients to move their legs occasionally during the times they're not exercising them. All patients should have properly applied antiembolic stockings (for example, TEDS) in place.

● *Monitor the patient's fluid intake and output.* If your patient is conscious and taking oral fluids well, his I.V. fluid intake may be limited to the amount he receives with the Amicar (aminocaproic acid) drip. (See page 77 for details.) If he's unconscious, increase the amount of I.V. fluids, as ordered, to keep him well hydrated.

When documenting your patient's fluid intake, remember to include any fluids he took with oral medications as well as any liquid oral medications, such as elixirs. Include your calculations on his intake and output flow sheet.

Nursing tip: If your patient must be catheterized — even intermittently — take precautions to prevent infection. Also, note the consistency, color, and odor of his urine each time you measure it. Call the doctor if you suspect urinary tract infection.

Chances are, the doctor has ordered a stool softener — and possibly a laxative — for the patient so he can move his bowels more easily. As you probably know, straining to defecate elevates intracranial pressure and may cause rebleeding. The use of stool softeners every day and laxatives periodically prevents this. *Caution:* Unless the doctor orders otherwise, never permit anyone to administer an enema to a patient with an aneurysm.

● *Feeding.* If your patient isn't fully conscious or can't swallow properly, the doctor may want him fed by nasogastric

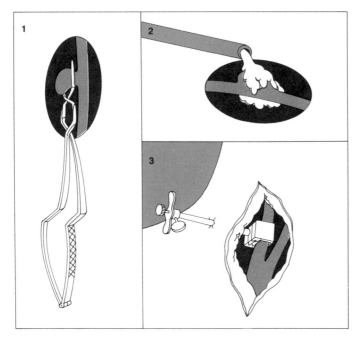

Surgery

For aneurysm patients, surgical treatment is the only sure method to prevent a rebleed. Here are the three procedures most commonly used:

Figure 1 shows a clip applied to the neck of an aneurysm. The clip may be one of several types, all of which are designed to exclude the defective area from circulation. Later, the arterial wall repairs itself, and the necrotic tissue detaches and is reabsorbed.

Figure 2 illustrates a procedure the doctor may use when an aneurysm site's inaccessible. The surgeon reinforces the aneurysm wall by wrapping it with:
• muscle, fascia, or other biologic material
• muslin or other types of cloth
• acrylic resins or other types of plastic.

Figure 3 shows placement of a carotid artery clamp, used to reduce blood pressure and flow within aneurysms of the internal carotid artery, or other aneurysms inaccessible to direct attack.

Following surgery, the doctor gradually tightens the clamp over a period of several days, thereby allowing time for collateral circulation to compensate for the reduced blood flow.

In caring for the patient at this stage of treatment, you should:
• Document how far the clamp is closed.
• Check neurologic signs every 5 to 10 minutes each time the clamp is tightened.
• Observe for weakness on contralateral side, and dysphasia (if left carotid clamped).
• Record temporal pulses with each neurologic check.
• Be sure handles to clamp are sterile and at bedside.
• Observe for possible infection; inspect dressing frequently.
• Position patient carefully to avoid pressure on dressing.

tube. However, if he can take oral liquids and food, observe these precautions: 1) Make sure he can swallow before you give him anything; 2) Never try to feed a patient or give him liquids while he's lying with his head flat. If you can't raise the head of his bed, attempt to feed him while he's lying on his side. (For more tips on how to feed that patient with facial weakness or other neurologic deficits, see Chapter 3.)

• *Eye Care*. Give eye care at least every 4 hours to any patient who has incomplete eye closure from facial weakness or loss of corneal reflex. To do this correctly, see Chapter 3.

The patient, his family, and you

Caring for the patient with a cerebral aneurysm is a nursing challenge. He's completely dependent on you and others for his physiologic needs. What's more, this dependency may be entirely new to him, because previously he may have been healthy. A ruptured cerebral aneurysm has a sudden onset — and may strike a person in his most productive years.

Coordinating all the treatment and care for this patient is your direct responsibility. This may be difficult, because he may need attention in many areas of the hospital. For example, you'll be working with health-team professionals in occupational and physical therapy, respiratory therapy, laboratory, and X-ray. You'll also be reporting to more than one doctor, especially if your patient has surgery.

Remember that a patient with a cerebral aneurysm may be left with neurologic deficits that frustrate, as well as embarrass, him and his family. Your positive attitude and encouragement will influence their response to these deficits and pave the way for a more satisfactory adjustment.

How long a patient must stay in the hospital after surgical repair of his aneurysm varies. Some patients need long rehabilitation or even transfer to a rehabilitation center. If not, your patient will need further care at home, which you'll have to take into consideration when you plan his discharge. And proper discharge planning always begins when the patient is admitted to the hospital, not on the day he's ready to leave for home.

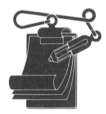

Remember these important points when caring for a patient with a cerebral aneurysm rupture:
1. Suspect this condition in a patient with neck stiffness, back and leg pain, fever, restlessness, irritability, occasional seizures, and blurred vision. These symptoms result from meningeal irritations caused by bleeding.
2. Be sure to establish and maintain an open airway, monitor neurologic status and record your findings, and provide bed rest with limited activity.
3. Be aware that surgical treatment of a cerebral aneurysm is the only way to prevent a rebleed.
4. Fit your patient with elastic stockings or Ace bandages immediately after admission, and apply them until he resumes activities. Remember, a patient with a cerebral aneurysm is particularly susceptible to pulmonary embolism.
5. Observe your patient for these life-threatening problems: rebleeding from the same site, vasospasm, pulmonary embolism, and hydrocephalus.

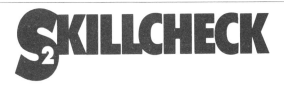

SKILLCHECK

Tom Crane is admitted to your unit with a diagnosis of CVA. He has right facial paralysis and right hemiplegia, as well as expressive aphasia.

1. When Mr. Crane was admitted to the emergency department, which of the following systems should have been evaluated first?
a) Respiratory
b) Cardiac
c) Neurologic
d) Genitourinary

2. Mr. Crane's facial paralysis may cause problems you'll want to prevent. Which of these may occur?
a) Corneal abrasion
b) Inability to open affected eye
c) Inability to swallow due to loss of gag reflex
d) Inability to talk

3. How do you position him to irrigate his mouth?
a) Supine, with his head elevated and facing forward
b) On his side with his right face uppermost
c) On his side with his left face uppermost
d) Supine with his head flexed forward

4. Based on his symptoms, Mr. Crane's lesion most probably is affecting his:
a) Right anterior cerebral artery
b) Basilar artery
c) Left posterior cerebral artery
d) Left middle cerebral artery

5. When you talk to Mr. Crane's family about his chance for neurologic improvement, what would you say is most characteristic of CVA?
a) There is usually no spontaneous recovery until several months after the stroke.
b) All stroke patients will have some chronic deficit.
c) Symptoms and recovery vary from one patient to another.
d) Spontaneous recovery is the only hope.

When Sally Wheeler is admitted to your unit from the emergency department, she's restless and confused. You note that all her extremities are strong and moving equally, and her pupils are equal and reacting. Several hours earlier she developed a severe headache and then later became confused. A lumbar puncture revealed bloody cerebrospinal fluid and an increase in pressure.

6. Why is Mrs. Wheeler placed on subarachnoid precautions?
a) To prevent her from falling out of bed
b) To insure that any change in her neurologic status will be reported immediately
c) To prevent any elevation in her arterial pressure, which may potentiate rebleeding
d) To provide her with complete nursing care.

7. Mrs. Wheeler has cerebral angiography done on the 5th day after admission and an aneurysm is detected on the right internal carotid artery. What specific neurologic findings might you find with a lesion in this area?
a) Weakness of the right arm and leg, dysphasia
b) Inability to look up or down with the right eye
c) Seizures
d) Enlargement and possible dilation of the left pupil.

8. Which of the following about Mrs. Wheeler's condition would make you call the doctor immediately?
a) Her rectal temperature rises to 100.2° F. (37.9° C.).
b) She refuses to cough vigorously.
c) She develops a sudden, new headache.
d) She remains confused.

9. Why did Mrs. Wheeler's doctor order that she receive aminocaproic acid I.V.?
a) To delay clot lysis, which can lead to rebleeding
b) To prevent pulmonary emboli
c) To prevent seizures
d) To prevent pulmonary edema.

(Answers on page 175)

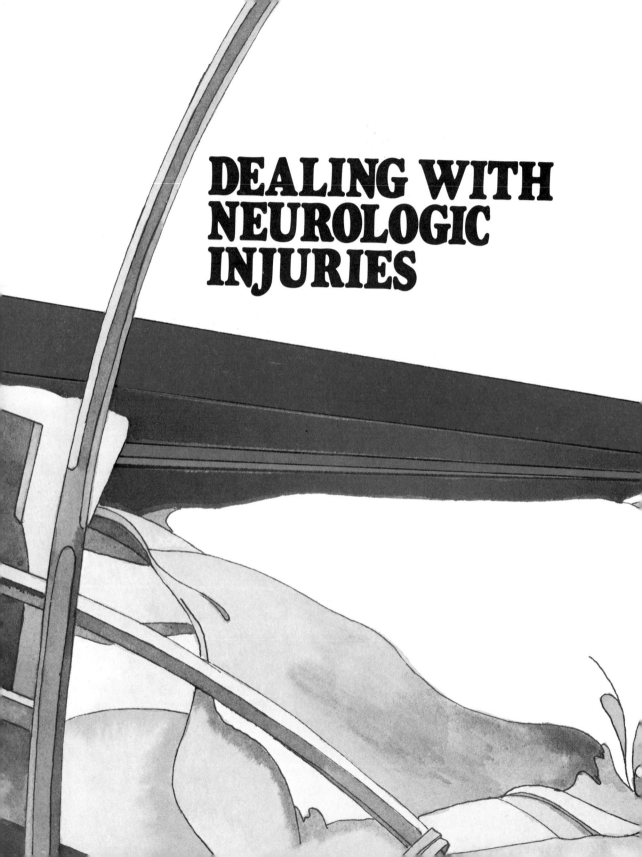

DEALING WITH NEUROLOGIC INJURIES

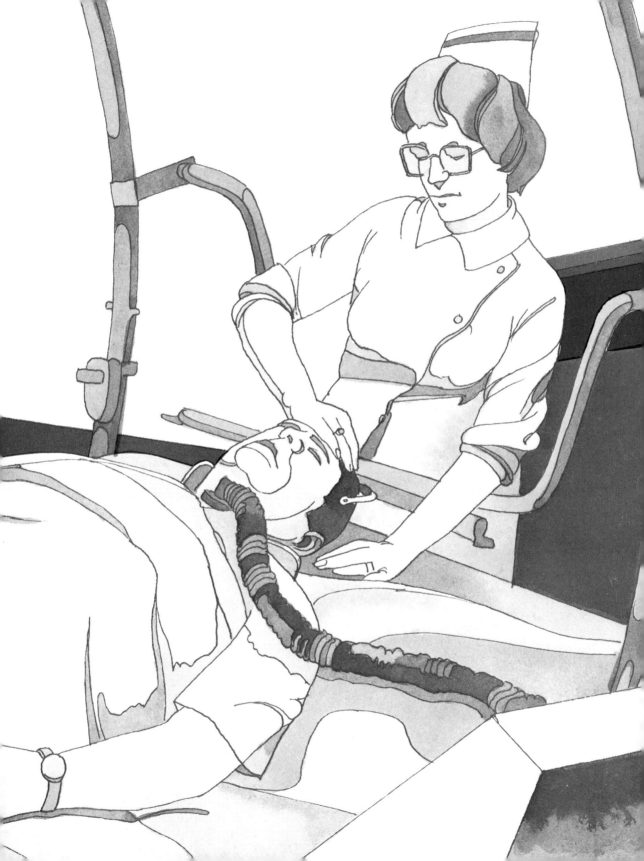

If you suspect your patient's intracranial
pressure is increasing, what
signs and symptoms should you look for?

Suppose your patient hit his head on a car
dashboard. What type of injury is likely?

What nursing actions can you take
to prevent your patient from experiencing
a sudden rise in ICP?

What areas of the spine are most
vulnerable to injury?

What complications frequently develop in a
patient with an injury above T8?

5

Head Injury
Preventing life-threatening complications

BY BARBARA KRAJEWSKI, RN

SHORTLY AFTER GALE WINDS whip through the resort area
where you work, your hospital's emergency department is
swamped with accident cases. The first you see is Richard
Black, a 22-year-old bartender, who has a head injury. According to police, he lost control of his car during the storm and
plunged down a 20-foot embankment.

You're told that Mr. Black lost consciousness for a short
time after the accident, but now he's awake and breathing
spontaneously. However, you notice that he seems unduly
agitated and doesn't realize he's in a hospital. "I don't think he
remembers the accident," the ambulance driver tells you.
"He's kind of confused."

What do you do next? Do you know what kind of emergency
care Mr. Black needs? How do you assess a head-injured
patient? Do you know how to position him properly? What
about his confusion? Suppose he later becomes combative?
What complications can occur with head injury? How can you
prevent them?

In this chapter, I'll give you the answers to all these questions. Then you'll know exactly what to expect the next time
you care for a patient like Mr. Black. I'll also explain why

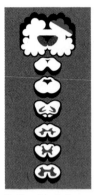

Pathophysiology
Cerebral injury results from either penetration or impact, which produces differential movement of the skull, brain, and meninges because of the varying masses of these structures. Damage may be caused by direct injury, or may be secondary to compression, tension, or shearing forces from the injury.

Head injury may also produce secondary phenomena such as ischemia and cerebral edema. Any of these, or a combination, can create a rise in intracranial pressure that further complicates the management of the injury. You can find an explanation of several types of head injury on page 88.

increased intracranial pressure sometimes occurs after head injury, and how it's measured. You'll learn about the current techniques used for intracranial pressure monitoring, as well as something about the risks.

Inside the skull

But first, let's talk more about the types of head injuries and how they affect the brain. As you probably know, when a patient's admitted with head injury, your main concern isn't the condition of his skull or scalp, but the condition of his brain and the degree of damage done to it. If you study the illustrations and text on page 88, you'll get some idea of what can happen inside a patient's skull when it's injured. A lot depends on the type of injury he receives: coup-contrecoup or acceleration-deceleration.

To understand what occurs when a person receives a coup-contrecoup injury, let's imagine a repairman falling down someone's basement steps and hitting his head on the cement floor. The blow bruises his brain and lacerates blood vessels just beneath the site of the trauma as his skull strikes against it. Then, as the transmitted blow drives the full force of the brain's weight to the opposite side of his head, contrecoup injury may follow. During this time, additional hemorrhages may occur where the brain strikes the bony prominences of the skull, such as the sphenoidal ridges.

Now let's see what happens inside a person's skull when he suffers an acceleration-deceleration injury. To illustrate, consider your patient Richard Black, as he plunges down an embankment and hits a tree. First, his head gets hurled forward, then snaps backward as his car comes to a halt. Inside the skull, his brain rebounds against bony ridges, resulting in bruises and lacerations of blood vessels.

When blood vessels in the brain are damaged, the blood may collect beneath the dura mater, forming a subdural hematoma; between the skull and the dura mater, forming an epidural hematoma; or within the brain's substance, forming an intracerebral hematoma. To help you review the differences between these complications and the symptoms they cause, I've listed them below:

• *Subdural hematoma:* An accumulation of blood usually from a torn vein on the brain's surface; most commonly found over the frontal and temporal lobes, where it may affect motor and language centers. Since blood accumulation from a venous bleed usually forms slowly, a patient may not develop symptoms suggesting hematoma for days or even weeks after the head injury. Watch for: depressed level of consciousness, seizures, and motor weakness or paralysis on one or both sides.

To remove a subdural hematoma, the doctor usually aspirates it through a burr hole.

• *Epidural hematoma:* A rapid, though rare, accumulation of blood between the skull and dura mater, usually caused by damage to the middle meningeal artery. The patient with this type of hematoma is usually unconscious immediately after the injury, then lucid for a short interval. Then the patient loses consciousness again from the accumulation of a large clot in the epidural space. Because the presence of this mass can affect cranial nerves, the patient may show the following signs and symptoms (on the same side as the lesion): pupil dilation and, as his condition deteriorates, facial weakness or paralysis. The patient needs immediate surgical aspiration of the hematoma to remove the mass and, hopefully, save his life.

• *Intracerebral hematoma:* An accumulation of blood within the brain's substance, usually from laceration or contusion of the frontal or temporal lobes. The patient's signs and symptoms vary, depending on the injury's location (see Chapter 4).

• *Tentorial herniation:* This occurs when injured brain tissue swells and forces itself through the tentorial notch. This squeezes the brain stem, affects vital centers and cranial nerves, and reduces the brain's blood supply. Symptoms vary. Watch for: drowsiness, confusion, dilation of one or both pupils, change in respirations, nuchal rigidity, bradycardia and — in late stages — decortication or decerebration. Be alert. Irreversible brain damage and death come quickly.

Assessing Richard Black

Now let's get back to your patient Richard Black who, according to reports, suffered an acceleration-deceleration head injury. He's conscious and breathing spontaneously when you see him first, but he's agitated and confused. A slightly lacerated arm is his only other apparent injury.

What do you do first? Here's a list of priorities to follow with any head-injured patient:

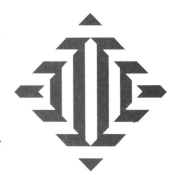

Danger signals
Any of these conditions in patients with head injuries may indicate a serious, perhaps life-threatening, situation:
• Deteriorating level of consciousness
• Onset of vomiting
• Changes in pattern of respiration
• Pupils — sluggish reaction to light. May progress to unilateral dilatation
• Developing hemiparesis.

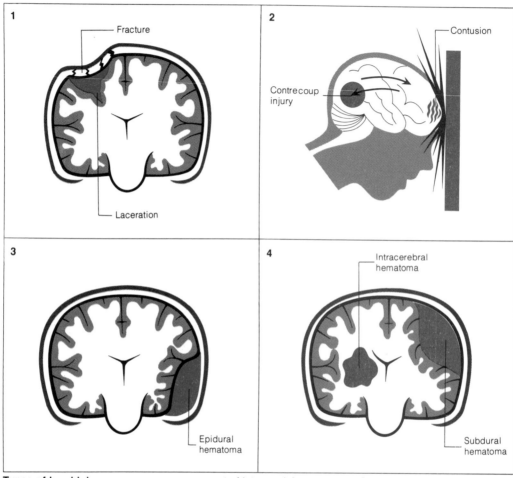

Types of head injury

Skull fracture. Fractures may be open or closed, depending on the integrity of the scalp. Laceration of the dura is apt to occur in an older patient, whose dura adheres more closely to the skull.

Laceration. May result from skull fractures or from brain striking irregularities of skull.

Contusion. Bruising of the cerebral cortex may occur at site of fracture particularly with depression or deformity of skull; also may result from a mass movement of intracranial contents against surface irregularities within the skull.

Rebound of the intracranial contents may occur opposite point of impact, producing *contrecoup* injury.

Epidural hematoma. Produced by hemorrhage into space between inner table of skull and dura. Temporal lobe is forced downward and inward, possibly causing uncal herniation; death may result. Usually associated with linear skull fractures, particularly of parietotemporal area.

Subdural hematoma. Produced by hemorrhage into potential space between the arachnoid and dura membranes. May follow contusion or laceration of the brain, or tearing of the veins bridging the subdural space.

Intracerebral hematoma. Usually associated with perforating or penetrating wounds involving laceration or contusion of brain substance.

Concussion. Transient state of unconsciousness following trauma, with apparent full recovery.

• Make sure he has an open airway and is breathing adequately. A head-injured patient with an obstructed airway may die from suffocation before he dies from damage to his brain. Clear his mouth and nostrils of debris, if necessary, but don't suction his nostrils until the doctor says it's okay. Nasal suctioning may induce leakage of spinal fluid through the nearby cribriform plate.

• Position your patient correctly, but make sure a cervical fracture has been ruled out by X-ray before you flex his back or neck. Never place a head-injured patient on his back; put him far over on either side. This prevents his tongue from occluding his airway and allows natural drainage of secretions.

Caution: Whenever you care for a head-injured patient, never place his head lower than the rest of his body. Doing so would increase pressure on his brain and possibly lead to herniation. But what if he's in hypovolemic shock, which may develop from concurrent injuries? Follow this procedure: Keep the patient's head flat or elevated, as before, but raise his limbs as much as possible to increase venous return to his heart.

• Find out all you can about the accident that caused his head injury. Get a complete description of what happened and try to learn if your patient lost consciousness at any time. (Of course, if your patient is groggy when you first see him, you may have to get the information from a witness.)

Try to learn if your patient was drinking or taking drugs before his accident. Ask when he ate last, so you'll know if he's likely to vomit and possibly aspirate the vomitus. The doctor may want you to insert a nasogastric tube to prevent this.

Gather as much information as you can about your patient's personal and medical history in the E.D. But if data *is* missing, be sure to document that *it is*. Then you or someone else can get it later when the information's available.

• Do a complete neurologic assessment as described in Chapter 2. Pay particular attention to level of consciousness and pupillary and motor responses. Watch for signs of increasing intracranial pressure (see pages 92 to 95).

• Check for concurrent injuries and possible cardiac problems.

• Check for bladder distention. The doctor may want you to insert a Foley catheter or start intermittent catheterization.

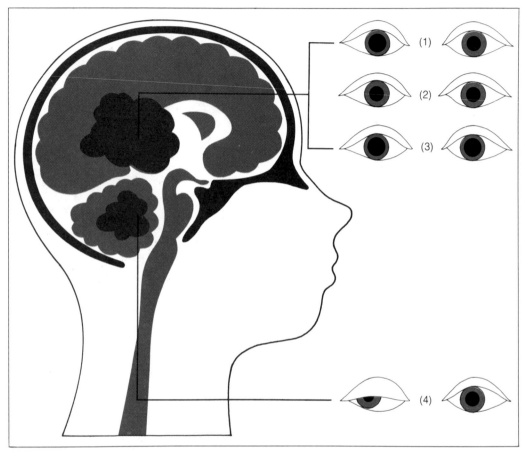

Identifying lesion site by pupillary signs

When you observe a patient with known or suspected cerebral injury, check for pupillary abnormalities. The type of abnormality is a convenient indicator of the lesion site.

As you know, pupillary constriction responses are controlled by the oculomotor (third cranial) nerve. An increase in intracranial pressure with herniation of brain tissue results in compression of this nerve. And because the *pupilloconstrictor* fibers run along the top of the nerve, they're compressed first.

When you examine the pupils, note relative sizes first and then test how the pupils react to light in a darkened room. When the lesion is in one hemisphere, the ipsilateral pupil may remain dilated and unresponsive to light level changes. Eventually, however, both hemispheres are affected by increasing cerebral pressure, and both pupils then remain fixed and dilated.

Supratentorial lesions:

Watch for differences in response to light. Remember, unilateral pupillary dilatation (1) generally occurs ipsilateral to lesion.

In later stage of midbrain compression, the pupils become fixed, and the eyes immobile (2).

Bilateral dilatation (3) indicates upper brain stem damage has already become extremely advanced.

Infratentorial lesions:

With cervical, sympathetic lesion, pupils are unequal, usually fixed. Horner's syndrome may be present. Watch for ptosis; ipsilateral pupillary constriction (4); decreased sweating on same side of face; enophthalmos (sinking in) of eyeball.

• Chances are the doctor will want you to start an I.V. with a fluid restriction to prevent further cerebral edema.

Whether or not your patient will be admitted to the hospital for further observation depends on how serious his head injury is. To determine this, the doctor will probably order these tests: X-rays of the skull, spinal column, and chest; EKG; EEG; and a computerized axial tomogram (CAT scan). He'll also want the patient to have a complete blood workup, including tests to measure arterial blood gases, electrolytes, and possible drug or alcohol ingestion.

Richard Black's tests were all within normal limits. His doctor diagnosed his head injury as a concussion. However, to be perfectly sure Mr. Black would receive prompt treatment if complications developed, he had him admitted to the hospital.

Continuing care for Mr. Black

Naturally, the doctor will continue to want frequent checks of Mr. Black's vital signs and neurologic status as long as he's in the hospital.

Watch for changes that indicate Mr. Black's condition may be deteriorating, and report them to the doctor promptly. Your biggest concern will be watching for signs of increasing intracranial pressure, preventing it if possible, and dealing with it if it occurs. For complete details on this important responsibility, see pages 92 to 95.

Nursing tip: Whenever you check your patient's neurologic status, document your findings exactly on the patient's assessment sheet or progress notes. Be specific, so you or others can make data comparisons later. For example, indicate exact pupil size by using a diagram that shows pupil gradations.

• Check for spinal fluid leaks, which may occur in a patient with a head injury, though infrequently. If you see fluid leaking from his ears and nose, immediately elevate his head 30° and call the doctor.

What else must you remember when your patient has a spinal fluid leak? Make sure he stays in bed and warn him not to lower his head. Suppose fluid is leaking from his nose. Carefully place a 4″ x 4″ gauze square underneath the nostrils so they can drain naturally. Advise him not to blow his nose, but to just wipe it. If fluid is leaking from an ear, position your patient so that his ear can drain and place a gauze square underneath it. (Continued on page 96.)

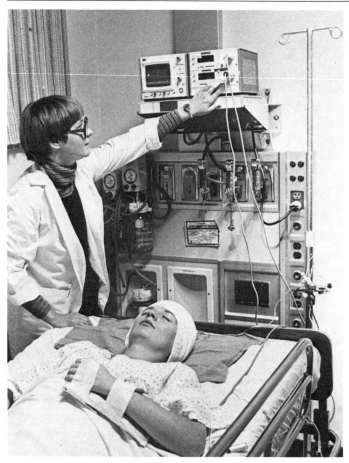

To prevent a sudden rise in ICP
- Maintain fully patent airway.
- When you must perform procedures that may elevate ICP (such as suctioning or changing positions), schedule them well apart to avoid compounding their effects.
- Maintain adequate ventilation:
  Monitor blood gases.
  Auscultate chest.
  Suction if necessary for 15 seconds maximum.
  Provided the doctor says it's okay, hyperventilate with O_2 before suctioning.
- Position carefully:
  Avoid prone position.
  Prevent neck flexion.
  Avoid extreme (90° or greater) hip flexion.
  Elevate head 15° to 30°.
- Prevent Valsalva's maneuver:
  Use stool softeners.
  Avoid enemas.
  Instruct alert patient to exhale while turning, moving in bed.
- Prevent isometric muscular contraction:
  Assist patient to move up in bed.
  Instruct patient not to push against foot board.
- Perform passive ROM exercises.

What causes ICP symptoms?
Cellular hypoxia. If ICP approaches or exceeds the mean systemic arterial pressure, the brain can't become adequately perfused and the cells become hypoxic. This, as you know, can lead to brain damage or death.

Brain shift or distortion
The only escape route for a swollen brain is through the tentorial notch. Pressure from an expanding mass (blood or tumor) may push structures out of midline. This results in compression of neurons and nerve tracts. As the displaced brain tissues compete with the brain stem for space in the

Intracranial pressure
As you know, the cranial contents — blood, brain, and cerebro-spinal fluid — are enclosed in a nearly inexpansible box, the skull.

Compensation
If the volume of any one of the cranial contents increases *slightly,* the brain can compensate by reducing the volume of one of the others slightly. For example, CO_2 retention during normal sleep produces cerebral vasodilation. This increases blood volume and

raises ICP. To compensate, the brain reduces intracranial CSF volume, thus returning ICP to normal.

Decompensation
The brain has only a small margin of compensation. Therefore, an *excessive* increase in volume will quickly exhaust its ability to compensate and ICP will rise. At the point when ICP has already increased, even a minor increase in volume can produce a major rise in ICP. By preventing those small increases, you can avoid a life-threatening situation.

Monitoring Intracranial Pressure

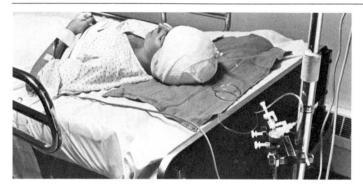

tentorial notch, the classic signs and symptoms of brain stem compression will appear:
• decreased LOC from impaired reticular activating system
• change in pupil size, equality, and extraocular movements, indicating impairment of the third, fourth, and sixth cranial nerves
• change in motor response (including onset of hemiparesis, decorticate or decerebrate posturing), indicating cortical or midbrain compression of motor tracts.
• changes in vital signs and pattern of respirations (which occur late), indicating great pressure on lower brain stem (pons and medulla).

When to monitor ICP
The doctor may decide to monitor ICP when your patient has intracranial hypertension from:
• an obstruction of his CSF circulation
• a space-occupying lesion
• cerebral edema.

How ICP monitoring works
First, the doctor implants a device to allow access to intracranial pressure. This pressure generates mechanical impulses which are picked up by a transducer and converted into electrical energy. This energy, in turn, is transmitted to a recording instrument and converted to visible wave forms

which appear on a chart recorder or oscilloscope. You'll be observing these wave forms for indications of increased intracranial pressure.

Signs and symptoms
Only a few of the classic signs of increased ICP occur early and then only at peak pressures.
As plateau waves begin, you may see subtle changes in the patient's level of consciousness, increased restlessness, and disorganized motor behavior (such as plucking at the bedcovers). The patient may complain of headache; he may seem less mentally acute. Changes in pupillary, motor, or vital signs (widening pulse pressure, slowing heart rate, irregular or decreased respiratory rate) occur more frequently at sustained peaks of pressure, not as the pressure rises. Don't wait until you observe them before you make a report.

Treatment
May include administering any of these medications:
• *Osmotic diuretics,* such as Mannitol, I.V., via drip or bolus, which is thought to reduce cerebral edema by shrinking intracranial contents. Remember, patients can become dehydrated very quickly, so monitor serum electrolytes and osmolality

closely. Be aware that a rebound increase in ICP may occur.
Tip: Store Mannitol at room temperature to avoid crystallization.
• *Steroids* lower increased ICP by reducing sodium and water concentration in the brain. May produce peptic ulcer, so they're usually given along with antacids and Cimetidine. Observe for possible GI bleeding.
• Barbiturates to induce coma, depressing the reticular activating system and allowing the brain to rest. With reduced demand for oxygen and energy, cerebral blood flow decreases, thereby lowering ICP.
Other treatments include:
• Fluid restriction, to avoid causing or increasing cerebral edema. Usually 1500-ml maximum per day.
• Hyperventilation with oxygen via Ambu bag or respirator. Helps the patient to blow off excess CO_2. A lowered PCO_2 constricts cerebral vessels, reducing cerebral blood volume and ICP.
• Measures to reduce temperature, in case of temperature elevation. Hyperthermia, as you know, increases brain metabolism. When cerebral blood flow increases to meet added demands for glucose, protein, and oxygen, ICP rises and creates a need for cooling. Measures include: administration of acetaminophen (Tylenol), alcohol sponge baths, hypothermia blanket. (For a discussion of nursing care when your patient is on a hypothermia blanket, see page 167).
The following procedures are less commonly used:
• The doctor may remove CSF either from the ventricle or by lumbar puncture; or he may surgically remove a bone flap to allow for brain expansion (temporal decompression).

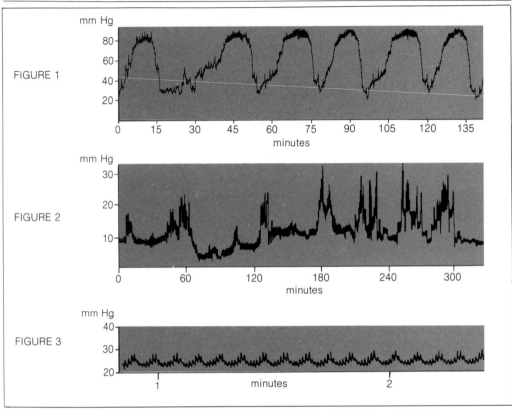

FIGURE 1

FIGURE 2

FIGURE 3

Interpreting ICP waveforms

As the illustration shows, the horizontal axis measures time (usually in minutes); the vertical axis measures intracranial pressure (in millimeters of mercury). When observing actual waveforms on the monitor, pay particular attention to elevations in pressure, and to how long the pressure remains elevated.

Normal pressure. 0 to 10 mm Hg with an upper limit of 15 mm Hg is considered normal intracranial pressure. Remember, however, that ICP is not static and that elevation in itself is not detrimental. Everyday activity requiring Valsalva's maneuver can raise ICP as high as 100 mm Hg.

Three types of ICP waveforms.
Figure 1. Plateau or "A" waves indicate rapid increases in pressure to 50 to 100 mm Hg. They are *sustained* elevations lasting approximately 5 to 20 minutes and followed by a rapid decrease in pressure. Patients who already have an elevated ICP are more likely to develop them. *Plateau waves may indicate ICP decompensation. Report them to the doctor immediately.* Remember, the prognosis is usually grave for patients who sustain ICPs greater than 50 mm Hg for more than 20 minutes.
Figure 2. "B" waves. Peaked, sharp, rhythmic oscillations with a sawtooth pattern, thought to be related to changes in respiration.

They occur every ½ to 2 minutes. Pressure may increase as much as 50 mm Hg, but elevations are *not sustained.* B waves are not clinically significant, and you don't have to notify the doctor.
Figure 3. "C" waves, correlated to changes in blood pressure, take the form of smaller rhythmic oscillations. Although they also may reach abnormal levels, they are not sustained elevations. C waves are not clinically significant, and you don't have to report them to the doctor.

Nursing Tip: Whenever you perform a nursing measure that may increase ICP, such as suctioning, make sure that you mark the readout strip. If you don't have readouts, document such care in your nurse's notes.

Monitoring Intracranial Pressure

Intracranial pressure measurement techniques

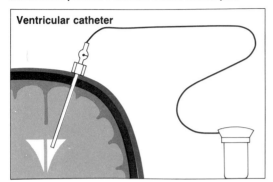

Ventricular catheter

Cannula and reservoir inserted into the brain's ventricle through a twist-drill hole in the skull.

ADVANTAGES
- Direct CSF measurement
- Access for CSF drainage sampling
- Access for determining volume-pressure responses
- Access for antibiotic installation.

DISADVANTAGES
- Risk of infection
- Difficulty in locating the lateral ventricles in a patient with midline shifting or collapsed ventricles
- Risk of brain tissue damage.

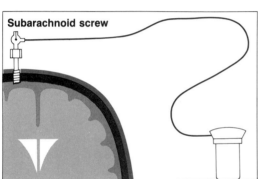

Subarachnoid screw

Steel screw with a sensor tip inserted through a twist-drill hole in the skull. Transducer attached to screw converts CSF pressure to electrical impulses.

ADVANTAGES
- Direct measurement from CSF
- Access for CSF drainage or sampling
- Access for determining volume-pressure responses.

DISADVANTAGES
- Risk of infection
- Requires skull firm enough to hold screw threads, as in patients over 6 years old
- Risk of screw plugging if skull swells.

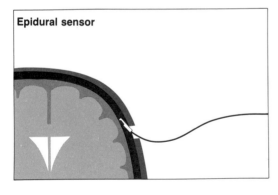

Epidural sensor

Tiny fiber-optic sensor inserted in brain's epidural space through burr hole in skull. Sensor cable plugs directly into monitor. Because this system cannot be recalibrated when affected by heat or pressure, its reliability remains controversial.

ADVANTAGES
- Less invasive.

DISADVANTAGES
- Questionable reflection of CSF pressure
- No route for CSF drainage
- Volume-pressure responses not feasible.

POINTS TO REMEMBER
- Irrigation is performed, when required, by the doctor.
- If you're assisting with irrigation, remember to use I.V. saline solution. *Never use the standard saline vials; they contain alcohol, which can cause cortical necrosis.*
- *Never use heparin:* The risk of small vessel bleeding is too great.

Never pack the ear canal to absorb fluid. Change and examine all dressings periodically and report your findings to the doctor.

Besides an ongoing neurologic check of Mr. Black's condition, the doctor may also order the following:

• complete bedrest with proper positioning and frequent turning

• restricted fluid intake to minimize cerebral edema, with accurate recording of urinary output

• medications, such as anticonvulsants and diuretics, given I.V. to prevent seizures and reduce the cerebral edema that may accompany head injury.

When concussion produces odd behavior

Even though Mr. Black escaped serious brain damage, his concussion produced a disturbing complication. Within a few hours, his behavior changed dramatically and he became very combative. He lashed out at those who were trying to help him and cowered on his bed like a trapped animal.

What caused him to act this way? To better understand, think back to Chapter 1 where you reviewed the functions of the temporal and frontal lobes. Now imagine how those functions may be disrupted if those portions of the brain are injured. You'll have a patient who becomes agitated, disoriented and confused, or a patient who suddenly starts acting like Mr. Black did, misinterpreting the actions and words of those around him.

Coping with the combative patient

What should you do in a case like this? And what shouldn't you do? Here are some helpful guidelines:

• Avoid using restraints, if possible. Restraining a patient with a head injury may cause even more damage, because it can elevate his blood pressure and thus increase intracranial pressure.

• Never sedate a head-injured patient, because sedation interferes with an accurate assessment of his level of consciousness. Sedation may also cause respiratory depression, which will increase the accumulation of carbon dioxide in the patient's bloodstream. (As you know, carbon dioxide is a powerful cerebral vasodilator. An abnormal accumulation of it can increase cerebral edema and intracranial pressure.)

• Speak to your patient in a gentle, reassuring voice, and continue to show that you care for him. This may not be easy to do if he's striking out at you verbally and physically. However, remember that he's confused because of his injury and probably frightened by the strange environment of the hospital. He may think you are trying to hurt him, and lashing out is his way to cry for help.

• Never make an unexpected or rapid move toward your confused, head-injured patient. Don't touch him in a way that might be interpreted as restraining, such as holding his hands. However, don't stop touching him entirely. Because a gentle touch may be just what he needs to reassure him. Nonverbal communications are more readily perceived than verbal ones, so accompany your words with some physical contact.

• Try to orient your patient to surroundings by explaining where he is and how you are trying to help him. Encourage his family to visit, and to bring him a radio, TV, and calendar. However, explain his irrational behavior to his family lest they become distressed by his personality changes. Suggest they use the helpful guidelines I've just discussed, so they can better cope with the patient's unfamiliar behavior.

• Finally, when your patient's ready to be discharged from the hospital, make sure he gets an appointment for follow-up care. Not all patients recover completely from brain injury, and even those who do recover may have some lingering effects. The long-term consequences of brain injury are post-traumatic syndrome, organic brain damage, and posttraumatic epilepsy. (For more information about epilepsy, see Chapter 9.)

The head-injured patient: A nursing challenge

By now you've learned that the head-injured patient presents you with a real nursing challenge, no matter how slight his injuries are. Even though he may have little or no lasting brain damage, he'll still need considerable support and reassurance. To this kind of comfort, add the comfort afforded by prompt, effective physical care. Then you'll have the winning combination you need to help your head-injured patient recover satisfactorily and return home.

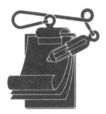

Remember these important points when caring for a patient with a head injury:
1. Be sure your patient has an open airway and is breathing adequately. This is always your first priority in providing emergency care for the head-injured patient.
2. Be alert for subtle changes in your patient's consciousness level as the first clue to increasing intracranial pressure.
3. Remember that your patient may not develop symptoms suggesting hematoma for days or even weeks after the head injury, because blood accumulation from a venous bleed inside the skull usually forms slowly.
4. After a head injury, check your patient's nose and ears for spinal fluid. If you notice spinal fluid, elevate the patient's head 30° and notify the doctor.
5. When the doctor irrigates an ICP measurement system, remember that he'll use I.V. saline solution. Standard saline solution contains alcohol and may cause cortical necrosis.

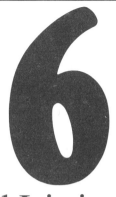

6

Spinal Cord Injuries
Coping with devastating damage

BY MARILYN PIRES, RN, MS

WHILE MAKING HIS ROUNDS in the intensive care unit, a neurosurgeon tells you to expect a new patient from the emergency department. The patient is 19-year-old Casey Doyle, who suffered a diving accident a few hours earlier. According to E.D. reports, he has a fracture dislocation of the fifth cervical vertebra, with spinal cord injury.

How do you prepare for Casey, who'll be arriving within the hour? You already know that he can't move his arms and legs, he can't feel sensations from the shoulders down, and he can't control his bowels and bladder. What kind of care will he need? What effect will his spinal cord injury have on each of his body systems? What life-threatening complications may occur? What are their danger signs? How will you react emotionally to such a devastating injury?

Caring for the patient who's suffered a serious spinal cord injury is surely one of the most difficult nursing challenges you'll ever face. His physical needs are almost overwhelming and require attention round-the-clock. His psychologic needs are heartbreaking, because — for a time at least — his injury may have left him helpless.

You can provide effective, supportive care to a patient like

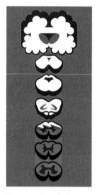

Pathophysiology
Most commonly, spinal cord
injuries result from trauma to the
spinal column, particularly when
displaced bone encroaches into
the spinal canal and compresses
the cord. However, even with little
or no bone injury, the cord may be
damaged by an interruption of its
blood supply. As you know, the
spinal cord's arterial system
doesn't have extensive collateral
circulation. Therefore, any
interruption of blood flow can
produce serious damage.
Trauma to the column may also
cause traction of the cord. Note,
however, that every injury to the
spinal column doesn't invariably
produce spinal cord damage.

Casey, no matter how serious his injury is. This chapter will
explain how, by outlining that care in detail. For example,
you'll learn how to prepare a patient for a Stryker frame and
how to keep him from being frightened once he's immobilized
on it. You'll also learn ways to make the patient on a Circ-
Olectric bed more comfortable, as well as the patient in skull
tongs.

What happens with spinal injury
Now let's take a closer look at spinal cord injuries and how the
level of injury affects a patient's muscle control. As you already know, complete injury to the spinal cord abolishes all
voluntary movement below the point of injury. Damage to
thoracic, lumbar, or (to some extent) the sacral cord segments
results in motor function loss of lower limbs: paraplegia. Damage to cervical cord segments results in some motor function
loss in upper limbs and total loss in lower limbs: quadriplegia.
To see exactly how these injuries affect specific motor responses in various parts of the body, see the opposite page
and page 102.

How does spinal cord injury affect a patient's sensory responses? In most cases, he'll immediately lose all sensory
function below the level of injury. For this reason, take care
that bath water, thermal blankets, and heating pads do not get
too hot. Otherwise, you may accidentally burn your patient
without his realizing it.

An exception to complete sensory function loss is hyperesthesia, in which the patient feels *abnormally increased*
sensations. Expect this patient to be hypersensitive to things
like light touch during bathing, water temperature, and bed-
linen weight.

Because spinal cord injury also affects the patient's autonomic nervous system, he may develop:

• orthostatic hypotension from loss of vasomotor control
below injury level

• inability to regulate his own body temperature, characterized by absence of sweating and shivering below injury
level

• neurogenic bladder and bowel.

For a complete description of the autonomic nervous system and how it works, see Chapter 1.

Of course, if a patient's cord is not completely damaged,

FUNCTIONAL GOALS IN SPINAL CORD LESIONS

SPINAL CORD LEVEL	MUSCLE FUNCTION	FUNCTIONAL GOALS
C3-4	Neck control: scapular elevators	• Manipulate electric wheelchair with mouth stick. • Limited self-feeding with ball-bearing feeders.
C5	Fair to good shoulder control; good elbow flexion	• Dress upper trunk. • Turn bed with arm slings. • Propel manual wheelchair with hand-rim projections or electric wheelchair with hand controls. • Self-feeding with hand splints. • Assist getting to and from bed.
C6	Good shoulder control; wrist extension; supinators	• Transfer from wheelchair to bed and auto with or without minimal assistance. • Self-feeding with tenodesis hands. • Assist getting to and from commode chair.
C7	Weak shoulder depression; weak elbow extension; some hand function	• Independent in transfer to bed, car, and toilet. • Total dressing independence. • Wheelchair without hand-rim projections. • Self-feeding.
C8 to T4	Good to normal upper extremity muscle function	• Wheelchair to floor and return. • Wheelchair up and down curb. • Wheelchair to tub and return.
T5 to L2	Partial to good trunk stability	• Total wheelchair independence. • Limited ambulation with bilateral long-leg braces and crutches.
L3 to L4	All trunk-pelvic stabilizers intact; hip flexors; adductors; quadriceps	• Ambulation with short-leg braces with or without crutches, depending on level.
L5 to S3	Hip extensors; abductors; knee flexors; ankle control	• No equipment needed if plantar flexion enough for push off at end of stance.

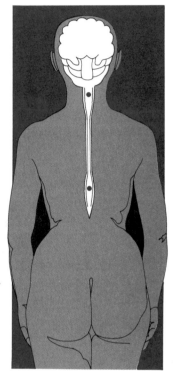

Vulnerable areas of the spine
Certain areas of the spinal cord are especially vulnerable to injury. Here's why:
• At the C5-C6 level, maximum movement of the cervical spine takes place. Besides that, the cord is enlarged at that level because of the many nerve fibers, which feed the upper extremities.
• A vulnerable back area is at the T12-L1 level. Again, maximum movement occurs here as well as an enlargement from the great number of nerve fibers feeding the lower extremities.
Below the spinal cord, the cauda equina floats within the vertebral canal. Mobility of these nerve roots inside the lumbar portion of the canal provides some measure of safety from injury.

Motor involvement in complete cord injury		
AREA OF VERTEBRAL INJURY	INVOLVEMENT	IMPLICATIONS
Cervical	Some degree of spastic quadriplegia. Intact reflex arcs below lesion after spinal shock, including bowel and bladder reflexes.	Possible severe contracture and mobility problems. Extensive rehabilitation needed. Automatic bowel and bladder activity possible with program.
Above C4	Paralysis of intercostals and diaphragm.	Respiratory failure, requiring assisted ventilation or phrenic pacing.
C4 and below	Paralysis of intercostals, although diaphragm functions.	Diaphragmatic self-breathing, but respiratory complications possible.
Thoracic	Some degree of spastic paraplegia. Intact reflex arcs below lesion after spinal shock, including bowel and bladder.	Possible lower contracture and mobility problems. Rehabilitation needed. Automatic bowel and bladder activity possible with program.
Lumbar and sacral	Flaccid paraplegia; flaccid bowel and bladder.	Possible lower contractures and mobility problems; some atrophy. Rehabilitation needed. Passive bowel and bladder activity possible with program.

some sensation and control may remain below the level of injury. How much of it remains — and in what combination — depends on the nature and position of the injury, as well as the patient's anatomic peculiarities.

Don't make things worse

As you know, when a person suffers spinal injury, most cord damage occurs at the time of the accident or in the handling shortly thereafter. Hasty and improper handling may cause the cord to be crushed, torn, pinched, or severed. That's why you must immediately immobilize a person with suspected spinal injury, *taking care not to move his neck or back.*

Fortunately for Casey Doyle, his diving accident was witnessed by friends trained in first aid. Instead of dragging him out of the water immediately, they kept him floating until they could place a board under him and carry him out. This technique reduced the chance of further injury to his spinal cord by providing firm support for head-neck-body alignment. (For further first aid tips should you witness an accident, see opposite page.)

Caring for Casey in the E.D.

Less than a half hour after his accident, Casey was transported by ambulance to the emergency department of a nearby hospital. Like most patients with spinal injuries, Casey was conscious, though pale and apprehensive. His vital signs were as follows: respirations, 24 and shallow; blood pressure, 80/40; pulse, 48; and temperature, 99°F. (37.2°C.).

Though you're a staff nurse in the intensive care unit, let's suppose you were working in the E.D. when Casey arrived on a stretcher. Turn back the clock a minute and imagine yourself on the scene. What do you do?

First, of course, you call the doctor. Then, before moving Casey from the ambulance stretcher, you and the other nurses follow these priorities:

• Make sure Casey has an open airway, and assess the rate and quality of his respirations. Anytime you care for a patient with a cervical injury, anticipate respiratory failure. Have the needed equipment ready in case the doctor has to perform a tracheostomy. He may prefer this procedure to endotracheal intubation, because he won't have to hyperextend Casey's neck.

Why is respiratory failure a special risk for Casey? First of all, his spinal cord was damaged at the C6 level, leaving C5 and above intact. This means he's lost the use of his intercostal and abdominal muscles and is breathing only with his diaphragm. This, of course, reduces his vital capacity, as well as the effectiveness of his respirations. In addition to this, he may have an accumulation of fluid in his lungs from the diving accident.

• If possible, keep Casey immobilized on the stretcher he came in on, until he's had all the X-rays and diagnostic tests he needs and his treatment has been decided. Take particular care not to move his neck. If a cervical collar wasn't applied at the accident site, apply one in the E.D.

Nursing tip: You can make a soft cervical collar by folding a towel around a 3"-wide piece of cardboard. For a newer method of immobilizing the neck, see the illustration on page 119.

Never try to move your spinal-injured patient before he's ready for transfer to another unit. Then don't attempt it unless you know how to do it properly and have enough people to help you (see page 146).

First aid
Suspect spinal cord injury in any patient with wounds of the face, neck, head, and shoulders, or in any patient unconscious from head injuries. Be alert for:
• paralysis of all extremities
• complaints of neck pain
• signs of spinal shock.

If any of these are present, don't move him without expert help, unless his life is in danger. As you know, improper handling can cause further damage to the cord.

First, assess the victim's breathing. If he needs artificial respiration, give mouth-to-mouth resuscitation using a modified jaw thrust. If this technique's unsuccessful, hyperextend his neck as a last resort to restore breathing. However, this procedure will almost certainly injure the cord further.

Should vomiting occur, carefully log-roll the patient — with enough help — to his side, keeping his head and neck aligned. Then, clear his mouth and throat with your fingers.

If he's conscious, reassure and protect him from further injury until the emergency vehicle arrives. In the ambulance, be sure his neck's immobilized, either with sandbags or with special immobilization devices some ambulances provide.

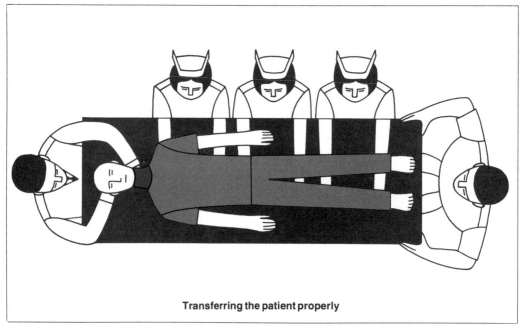

Transferring the patient properly

Transfer techniques

Move your spinal cord injured patient as little as possible. However, if you must transfer him to a bed or stretcher, follow these guidelines:
• Does your patient have a possible cervical injury? Don't move him until a neck immobilizer's in place.
• Enlist the help of at least four people to transfer your patient. Three should stand on the same side. The leader, preferably a doctor, stands at the patient's head to direct the transfer. When he says "lift," everyone must keep in line and lift together, taking care to maintain the patient's spinal alignment. Once's he's lifted, a fifth person standing at the patient's feet moves the stretcher safely out of the way. During this transfer, the leader may apply manual traction to the patient's head and neck.

• Assess Casey's condition by getting his history and asking him exactly how the accident happened. If he was unconscious or unable to answer questions, you'd get the information from his family or whoever accompanied him.

Now evaluate the extent of his injuries by doing a neurologic assessment, as described in Chapter 2. Casey's assessment indicates that he has shoulder control and elbow flexion, but no other voluntary motor functioning below the fifth cervical level. He can raise his arms at will, but he can't bring them down. When you see him, he has his arms raised — flexed at the elbows and wrists — and tucked under his chin. His pupils are equal and reacting to light. He has no lacerations or other indications of head injury.

Your sensory assessment of Casey indicates that he feels sensations in these three areas: his back (to just below the collar area); his chest (to just below the clavicle); and on both arms from shoulder to wrist (a strip of sensation on the upper third of the anterior surfaces). For a dermatome chart showing how you can chart your sensory assessment, see page 42.

• Anticipate spinal shock, which occurs inevitably when the cord's completely damaged. This condition lasts anywhere from a few minutes to a few weeks and can best be described as a neurovascular shutdown response to spinal trauma (see the discussion on this page).

To support the patient when spinal shock symptoms develop, the doctor will probably want you to start an I.V. with lactated Ringer's solution, insert a Foley catheter to prevent urinary retention, and insert a nasogastric tube to reduce gastric distention. Keep in mind that Casey's using his diaphragm to breathe because his other muscles are paralyzed. If you let gastric distention go unrelieved, it may press on his diaphragm and lead to respiratory arrest.

Another reason for inserting a nasogastric tube is this: It'll prevent aspiration of vomitus, if vomiting occurs.

Along with the lactated Ringer's solution that Casey's receiving, the doctor wants him to have a steroid, dexamethasone (Decadron) I.V., to reduce spinal cord edema. Casey has no pain at the injury site, so he doesn't need an analgesic. But if he did, the doctor would order a mild one, because anything potent, like morphine, could further depress respirations.

How is Casey's condition diagnosed?

Besides studying the information you've collected, the doctor has to evaluate the results of various diagnostic tests before he can determine Casey's treatment. For example, he'll need X-rays of Casey's entire spinal column to tell the extent of injury. X-rays must show all segments of the column, because the injury may involve more than one vertebra.

Besides spinal X-rays, Casey may require the following:
• a myelogram. This checks the flow of cerebrospinal fluid (CSF) and locates a blockage, if it exists. When normal flow of CSF is interrupted at any point, it indicates pressure on the patient's spinal cord. To relieve the pressure, he may require immediate surgery.
• arterial blood studies to measure blood gases
• vital capacity and tidal volume tests to evaluate respiratory functions
• chest X-ray, EKG, and routine blood studies.

What will the doctor decide?

As you already know from the beginning of this chapter, Casey's test results show that he has a fracture dislocation of the fifth cervical vertebra with a complete transection of his

Spinal shock

Immediately after spinal cord trauma, expect the patient to undergo a period of spinal shock, or *areflexia*, which is a sudden neurovascular shutdown response. Spinal shock can last from minutes to days, and in some cases as long as several weeks. During this period, watch closely for these problems:

• *Hypotension*, resulting from loss of vascular tone below injury level. You can distinguish it from hypovolemic shock by its associated bradycardia, rather than tachycardia.

• *Hypothermia or hyperthermia*, with no sweating below the injury level. Patient's temperature will be ambient.

• *Flaccid paralysis* below the injury level with bowel and bladder atony. Expect sacral reflexes and priapism, but only in patients with upper motor neuron lesions.

Note: In patients with upper motor neuron lesions, the end of shock is marked by the return of reflexes and by spasticity. Obviously, no reflex activity will return in patients with lower motor neuron lesions.

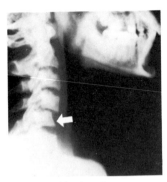

Evidence of a break
This spinal X-ray indicates a fracture dislocation of the 5th cervical vertebra. Such fractures are commonly associated with damage to the spinal cord.

spinal cord. Measurements of his blood gases, vital capacity, and tidal volume are abnormal, though not enough (at the time) for Casey to require assisted ventilation. The doctor sends Casey to the O.R. for placement of skull tongs, then on to the ICU for further treatment.

What treatment does the doctor plan for Casey? He decides on a conservative approach: 1 to 2 weeks in cervical traction to achieve alignment, then 8 to 12 weeks in a halo device. During the time Casey's in cervical traction, he'll remain in a regular hospital bed equipped with a traction frame and movable pulley. However, sometimes patients requiring skull traction are cared for on a Stryker frame. The skull tongs and Stryker frame aren't the only pieces of specialized equipment used to manage spinal injuries; there are others that you'll learn about later in this chapter.

Obviously, not all spinal-injured patients will receive the same treatment as Casey. Much depends on the type of injury, as well as its location. The goals of treatment remain the same, however: to save patient's life, protect the spinal cord from further damage, and provide an optimal environment for neurologic healing.

Here are some of the treatment possibilities open to the doctor:
• cervical traction applied with skull tongs or a halo device (for patients with cervical injuries)
• postural reduction in bed with no weight bearing on spinal column (for patients with thoracic-lumbar injuries)
• surgery — laminectomy, with or without fusion, or insertion of immobilization rods. (For more on these procedures, as well as the nursing care involved, see Chapter 8.)

What's your role?
No matter what the doctor decides to do, your role in caring for the patient with severe spinal injuries will be challenging. His physical needs are considerable and involve all areas of his body. You must understand how to assess him by system, and know what to look for. If you don't, he's apt to develop a life-threatening complication — or, if not that, one that may inhibit his chances for an optimal recovery.

When Casey reaches the ICU, continue the neurologic checks that were started in the emergency department. Take and record his vital signs frequently, keeping in mind that he'll still be in spinal shock. *Document all your findings without delay, and be very specific about details.* If you're not, no one will have an accurate baseline to compare subsequent changes to. (For information on how to document a patient's condition properly, read the Nursing Skillbook, DOCUMENTING PATIENT CARE RESPONSIBLY.)

As you continually check your patient's neurologic signs, carefully assess the degree of involvement. Does he show any change in reflexes, strength, sensations, or ability to move? *If he does, tell the doctor immediately and document your findings.*

Giving Casey respiratory care

Now let's talk about the attention you'll be paying to Casey's body systems, starting with your top priority: his respiratory system.

As you know, when Casey arrived in the E.D., he was breathing independently, using his diaphragm. However, if edema ascends above the C4 level, he may find his diaphragm getting paralyzed. This can happen anytime within the first 48 hours, so you must be ready for it.

Anytime you care for a patient like Casey, pay close attention to his breathing. Keep checking his blood gas measurements, which — in a stable, uncomplicated quadriplegic — are acceptable at these figures: PO_2, 60 mm Hg and CO_2, 45. Check his tidal volume, which under the same circumstance, is acceptable at 200 ml. Report any changes in these baseline figures immediately, especially if they're accompanied by changes in the rate, rhythm, or quality of respirations.

Respirations that suddenly become rapid and shallow with flaring of the nostrils are a bad sign. If you suspect trouble, ask the patient to count up to 30 without taking a breath. If he can't count up to 10 without taking a breath, call the doctor. Also notify him if you observe anxiety, cyanosis, or mental confusion.

Get help immediately if your patient begins to develop respiratory distress. If the doctor wants to perform a tracheostomy, prepare your patient for the procedure by explaining that it'll help him breathe again. Reassure him that you'll be checking him frequently. Remember, after he's had a tracheostomy performed, your patient will have no way to call for help.

Sense and sensitivity

When talking with your patient, do you sometimes use touch to communicate your concern for him? A touch on the hand may offer comfort and reassurance to the patient who's feeling isolated. Don't forget, however, that a spinal cord injured patient may lack sensation in his hands. Always determine where he has sensation, so you can reinforce your verbal messages of caring with a gesture he'll perceive, such as a touch on the forehead. Make sure you document his level of sensation in your nurses' notes to help others communicate with him meaningfully.

After your initial assessment, mark your patient's skin with a felt-tip marker to indicate where you're assessing sensation. Keep a dermatome chart (see page 42) near the patient's bed for reference when checking for sensory gains or losses. Be sure to document any observation along with the date and time. Report any sudden changes to the doctor immediately.

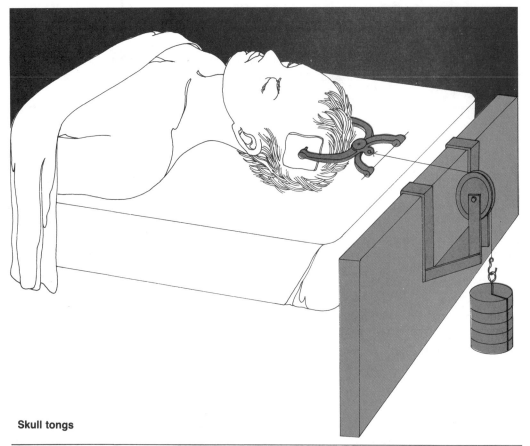

Skull tongs

How to care for the patient in skeletal traction

Typically, a patient whose spinal cord has been injured must be immobilized for some time, usually 4 to 12 weeks. How long depends on the level of his injury and the prescribed treatment.

Of course, whatever immobilization method the doctor prescribes for your patient, you'll want to understand the necessary equipment and care.

First, let's talk about skeletal traction for cervical injuries. Refer to page 116 for the care you'll give to a patient immobilized on a frame or bed. If your patient has a cervical injury, the doctor

may use skeletal traction.

Skull tongs

One form of skeletal traction is skull tongs (for example: Crutchfield, Barton, or Gardner-Wells). To insert Crutchfield tongs, the doctor will drill shallow burr holes over each parietal region. Next, he'll insert the tongs' points into the openings and apply a sterile dressing. (*Note:* Gardner-Wells and Barton tongs do not require burr holes and can be inserted in the E.D.) To provide traction, he'll extend a rope from the center of the tongs over a pulley and attach weights to the other end.

No doubt this procedure will

frighten the patient and his family. Ease their minds by explaining what the doctor will do in advance. Assure them that the tongs won't penetrate his brain, just the outer layers of his skull.

After the tongs are in place, maintain traction at all times. Make sure the rope doesn't get caught in the mattress and that the weights never rest on the floor. Don't release traction unless the doctor orders it. Then remove the weights gently. The doctor may want this patient cared for in a regular bed.

Here's how to care for your patient's tong site. Remove his dressing daily and inspect for

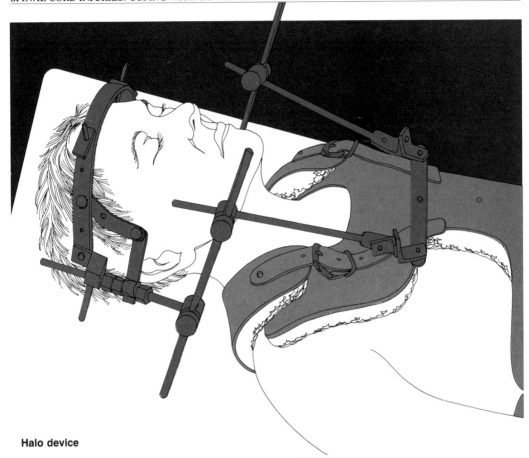

Halo device

Halo device

Another form of a skeletal immobilizer for patients with cervical
injuries is the halo device (see
above).

For this, the doctor places an
adjustable stainless steel hoop
around the patient's head and
secures it to his skull with two
occipital and two temporal
screws. Steel bars anchor this
device to the patient's body cast
or sheepskin-lined vest.

The halo allows your patient

signs of infection. Clean the site
with an antiseptic and apply a
sterile dressing. Report any signs
of infection to the doctor.   ,

greater mobility, with minimal risk
of disturbing his spinal alignment
during position changes. He's
usually permitted out of bed
earlier than a patient with skull
tongs because the alignment
can be maintained more easily.

You'll probably care for your
patient with a halo in a regular
hospital bed. Place him on either
side, as well as supine or prone.
Do not elevate his head or legs.
In the acute phase, you may
wish to avoid the prone position.
Not only does this position make
respiratory assessment more
difficult, but it may also disturb
the patient whose face is inches
away from the mattress.

Get assistance when changing
your patient's position every 2
hours. Use a pull sheet. Lift but
don't drag him to the side of
the bed. Then roll him to the desired position; never turn or lift
him by grabbing the halo.

If a pin becomes detached
from the halo, don't move the
patient. Call the doctor. Stabilize
the patient's head with your
hands until the doctor arrives.

Nursing tip: Your patient in
skull tongs or halo traction will
be especially sensitive to any
noise made by striking the metal
since bone is an excellent sound
conductor. Avoid letting anything
hit these metal devices.

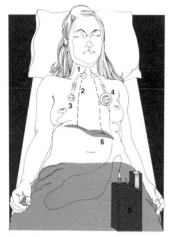

Keeping pace
Until recently, people with injuries above C4 were restricted by bulky respiratory equipment and the need for continual daily care. Now some patients have the opportunity to live more normally, thanks to the development of the phrenic nerve stimulator (diaphragm pacer).

Here's how it works: The doctor surgically implants an electrode (1) around each of the two phrenic nerves (2). Then he attaches each electrode to separate subcutaneous receivers. Over one receiver (3), he tapes an antenna (4) to the patient's skin and attaches it to a transmitter (5). This transmitter, when set, controls the rate and intensity of stimulation to the diaphragm (6). After 12 hours, and every 12 hours thereafter, the antenna is placed over the alternate receiver. In this way, each phrenic nerve has an active and a resting period.

If the doctor wants him to go on a respirator, give your patient the instruction he needs. For example, urge him to relax and not fight the machine. Your attitude can relieve his fear and anxiety more than almost anything else.

Naturally, you'll try to keep your patient from developing respiratory distress by giving him specialized care. Provided it's okay with the doctor, here are some guidelines you can follow when you're caring for a quadriplegic like Casey:

• Turn him every 2 hours.

• Make sure he has postural drainage at least once every shift, if he's immobilized in a way that makes this possible. After drainage, give him chest physiotherapy and help him cough, using the quad coughing method. To do this, place the palm of your hand under his diaphragm and push down forcefully when he exhales.

• Give regular intermittent positive-pressure breathing (IPPB) treatments to stretch his chest wall and prevent accumulation of lung secretions. This is especially important for quadriplegics like Casey, because they no longer can sigh.

• Suction only as needed, using strict aseptic technique.

One other important note on respiratory care for spinal-injured patients: Until recently, patients with injuries above the C4 level were doomed to a very limited life-style because they couldn't exist without bulky respiratory equipment and almost constant nursing care. Now, however, some of them can benefit from a portable ventilator, or the phrenic nerve stimulator, which is illustrated on this page.

What about your patient's gastrointestinal system?

For a time at least, a quadriplegic patient like Casey will have paralytic ileus from spinal shock. How long this condition will last varies. Keep checking for bowel sounds to return, or for the passage of flatus or stool. When paralytic ileus has disappeared, the doctor will probably want the patient to have his nasogastric tube removed and start on an oral diet.

Watch for symptoms of a stress ulcer somewhere between the 6th to 14th day after injury. You should call the doctor immediately if you see bleeding in the patient's stool or vomitus. (As you may know, this ulcer is thought to be caused by an abnormal release of stress hormones into the patient's system after injury. The condition is complicated by the steroid drugs that the doctor may have ordered for the patient when he was admitted to the hospital.)

You'll find it hard to detect a stress ulcer or other acute abdominal problem in a patient like Casey, because he won't feel pain below the level of his injury. In quadriplegics, be alert for a sudden, unexplained shoulder pain. It may be a referred pain, so report it to the doctor immediately.

After a time, your patient will be stable enough to have a regular bowel program. First, find out what his normal bowel habits were before his injury. Then try to establish a pattern close to that. If the doctor agrees, follow these guidelines: Insert a suppository in the patient's rectum, then use digital stimulation. If nothing happens within an hour, manually remove any stool present in the lower bowel. Repeat daily until a routine is established. Stool softeners, mild laxatives, sufficient liquids, and a diet adequate in roughage may help. If you see no results within 5 days, the doctor may order an enema. Then, reinstate the regular bowel program.

Preventing and caring for genitourinary problems

While your patient's in spinal shock, he'll need a Foley catheter because his bladder will be paralyzed. Maintain a closed, patent drainage system at all times. Give regular catheter care, use the taping techniques illustrated on page 112, and check for obstructions frequently.

Observe and document the patient's urinary output. Is he receiving I.V. fluids? The doctor may want you to titrate them to make sure he maintains an adequate output. However, remember that his output may be low at first because of hypotension from spinal shock. Titrate carefully, so you don't overload him with fluids, which can lead to pulmonary edema.

Later, if reflex activity returns to his bladder and fluid balance stabilizes, your patient may require intermittent catheterization. (Sometimes it's attempted immediately after the injury.) This helps maintain bladder tone and prevent urinary tract infections. If the doctor decides that your patient's a suitable candidate for intermittent catheterization, the first step may be to determine, through lab studies, whether he needs antibiotic or urinary antiseptic treatment. Next, begin a teaching program to familiarize the patient and his family with the anatomy and physiology of the urinary tract; the equipment and techniques of the procedure; principles of asepsis; and the importance of keeping accurate fluid intake and output

A critical complication

Autonomic dysreflexia or hyperreflexia is an emergency associated with spinal cord injuries. An uninhibited reflex response to a noxious stimulus, this syndrome may develop in patients with injuries above T8. It usually happens after the patient's over spinal shock; at a time when reflexes return and visceral tone's recovered. The first episode may occur anytime up to 6 years after injury.

Here's what happens: A noxious stimulus initiates an autonomic reflex action of total body vasoconstriction. Normally the body's compensatory vasodilation mechanism gets activated at this point, but now the lesion prevents most of the message from getting through. However, the message to slow the heart travels via the vagus nerve and causes bradycardia. If not interrupted, this cycle can cause seizures or stroke from severely elevated blood pressure; or cardiac arrest from continued bradycardia. Symptoms include:
• pounding, severe headache
• paroxysmal hypertension
• flushing above injury level, with pallor below level
• shivering and gooseflesh, followed by profuse sweating above injury level
• fast, bounding pulse, followed by progressively slowing pulse. Prevent the most common stimuli initiating dysreflexia: bladder distention, fecal impactions, or decubitus ulcers. If, despite your precautions, these symptoms appear, immediately elevate the patient's head, unless contraindicated, and relieve any bowel or bladder distention. If symptoms don't subside, call the doctor.

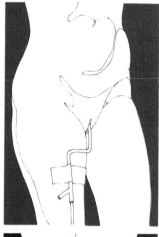

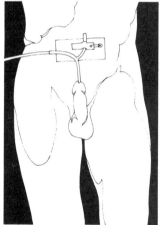

Catheter tip
Anchoring a Foley catheter as shown helps prevent accidental traction that could injure the patient's bladder or urethra. Anchoring it to the male patient's abdomen helps prevent penoscrotal fistula.

To do this, wash and dry a 4-inch area on the upper thigh (or abdomen for males). Shave if hair growth is heavy. Apply a 4-inch piece of tape around catheter, then to skin on either side.

Leave enough slack in the catheter to keep tape from causing tension.

records. In setting up an intermittent catheterization program, remember that fluid intake and elimination must always be balanced. No more than 600 ml of urine should accumulate at any time. As you know, overdistention destroys the detrusor muscle's ability to contract, thereby jeopardizing return of automatic function after spinal shock. Besides, it may weaken the antireflux mechanism at the vesicoureteral junction, endangering the upper urinary tract.

The procedure itself begins with catheterization every 4 hours. After observing the patient's elimination patterns, adjust the interval between catheterizations accordingly. First, try to elicit spontaneous voiding by stimulating his sacral reflex arc (thigh-stroking), or doing Credé's method, depending whether his lesion's upper or lower motor neuron. If he's successful in voiding, catheterize him afterward to obtain a residual. Discontinue catheterizations when residuals are less than 150 ml. However, for the patient who can't void spontaneously, continue planned interval catheterizations.

If your patient's physically and mentally capable, begin teaching him self-catheterization. Make sure he understands the need to limit his evening fluid intake. By doing so, he'll avoid overdistending his bladder and interrupting his sleep for catheterizations.

Complications in the cardiovascular system
Expect a patient like Casey to have various cardiovascular problems because of his injury. That's why he'll be on an EKG monitor in an ICU, so you can detect difficulties early.

During spinal shock, vasomotor tone is lost, blood pools in the capillaries, and the circulating volume shrinks. Expect hypotension and bradycardia.

You may also see orthostatic hypotension, because the patient can no longer compensate for position changes. This occurs because the vasoconstricting message from the medulla can't pass the damaged cord and reach blood vessels.

Because of this, your patient may faint when you turn him on a Circle bed. If this happens, don't waste time analyzing the situation. Continue turning to get him to a flat position. Later, when his condition permits, the doctor may want you to gradually elevate his bed. Check his vital signs every 5 minutes. At first, even the slightest elevation may cause his blood pressure to drop dramatically. If this happens, return the patient to a flat position and try again later. Gradually, he may be able to tolerate increased elevation. You may also want to apply an abdominal binder, antiembolism stockings, or Ace bandages on the patient's legs to increase venous return.

Thrombosis is another problem that's likely to occur because of your patient's compromised cardiovascular system. To help prevent it, apply antiembolism stockings to his legs and start passive range-of-motion exercises. Some doctors may also order low doses of heparin prophylactically. *Nursing tip:* Remember, your spinal-injured patient won't feel the pain that usually accompanies thrombosis. So don't wait for him to complain of it. Instead, watch closely for redness or swelling in his legs, and, if they appear, notify the doctor. Measure the patient's legs once each shift and mark where you measured. Document it.

Meeting your patient's nutritional needs

As soon as your patient is over spinal shock, the doctor will probably want him to start on a high-calorie, high-protein diet. Making sure he stays with this diet may be difficult, but it's important. A patient with a spinal injury tends to lose weight easily, because of the increased catabolic activity that accompanies his injury.

Chances are, your patient isn't going to have much of an appetite — partly because he's depressed, and partly because he's suffered sensory loss. Do everything you can to help restore his pleasure in eating. For example, encourage his family to bring his favorite foods from home. Send out for hamburgers or pizza from a fast-food chain. Or ask the dietary department to supply between-meal milk shakes.

Give good skin care

You'll find nursing orders for good skin care on the care plan for every patient, but particularly the one who has a spinal injury. As you know, the spinal-injured patient may be immobilized for up to 12 weeks. He'll need meticulous attention to keep him from developing those pressure-reddened areas that easily become decubitus ulcers.

To give your patient good skin care, use these guidelines:
• Change his position at least once very 2 hours. Besides preventing pressure areas, this also prevents contractures and

Danger signals
Any of these conditions in patients with spinal cord injuries may indicate a serious, perhaps life-threatening, situation.
• Increased loss of sensation
• Increased loss of motor functioning
• Severely pounding headache associated with hypertension
• Changes in patterns of respiration.

respiratory complications (For information on how to turn a patient who's immobilized by such special equipment as skull tongs, see pages 108 and 109.

• Use incontinence pads rather than a bedpan when you give routine bowel care. A bedpan doesn't work well for three reasons: It's so hard it can cause a pressure area over your patient's coccyx; it doesn't allow easy access to the anus for digital stimulation; and it can upset the spinal alignment necessary for proper healing. *Important:* Don't use incontinence pads continuously, just during bowel care. The pads retain moisture and can cause skin breakdown.

• Keep the patient's skin clean and dry, especially where there are folds with skin-on-skin contact. Add bath or mineral oil to the bath water to help prevent skin cracking. Pay special attention to the patient's feet. To remove calluses and scaliness from heels and soles, do the following: Wash feet and apply lanolin generously; wrap warm moist towels around each foot; encase each foot in a plastic bag for 1 to 2 hours; remove bag and towels; and gently peel away dead skin. Repeat as needed.

For further information on how to keep your patient's skin clean and intact, read the rehabilitation feature in Chapter 3.

Prevent contractures
Don't wait till your spinal-injured patient gets past the acute stage before you attempt to prevent contractures. Connective tissue changes from disuse can produce muscle shortening within 3 days. What's more, the muscles a patient uses to *flex* an extremity are stronger than those he uses to *extend* it. So his paralyzed extremity is more likely to contract in a flexed position (once it's there), then an extended position.

If allowed to develop, contractures will seriously limit your patient's ability to make an optimal recovery. For example, hand and arm contractures may keep him from feeding, dressing, and grooming himself. They may also keep him from using hand splints or other adaptive devices that could give him greater independence.

Leg and feet contractures can also be devastating. If allowed to develop, they may: interfere with your patient's comfort in a wheelchair; keep him from wearing shoes or leg braces; complicate dressing and perineal hygiene; and limit positions for sexual activity.

To prevent contractures, keep your patient properly

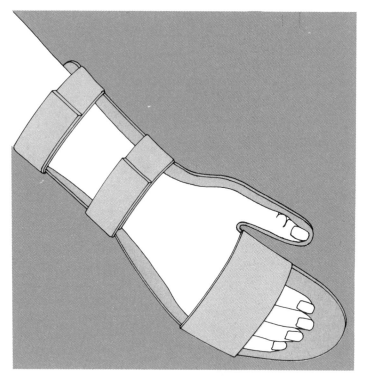

A practical application
You may apply splints to your patient's paralyzed wrist and hand to prevent wristdrop and maintain a functional arm position. You may also apply a variation of this splint that keeps the thumb in opposition. (See illustration.)

To help prevent skin breakdown sometimes caused by splints, apply the splints for 2 hours, then remove them for a 2-hour period. Indicate this rotation schedule on the patient's care plan. For easier management, tailor his splint care to fit his turning schedule.

positioned with pillows; Spenco boots; and leg or hand splints (see above). Work in cooperation with the physical and occupational therapy departments to write out a plan of care. Don't use sandbags in your patient's bed, because these can cause skin breakdown. Avoid rubber doughnuts, because they restrict circulation, leading to increased edema.

Passive range-of-motion exercises also help prevent contractures. To learn more about these, plus the various positioning devices listed above, see Chapter 3.

Give psychologic support early

Up to now, I've talked only about the physical care your patient needs. However, don't be so overwhelmed by it that you neglect his psychologic needs. Try to imagine what life is like for the quadriplegic. He can't move or feel anything from the neck down. He sees little of his surroundings, especially if he's immobilized by skull tongs. He may not even be able to communicate as he wishes, if he has a tracheostomy.

Turning your patient on a Stryker frame

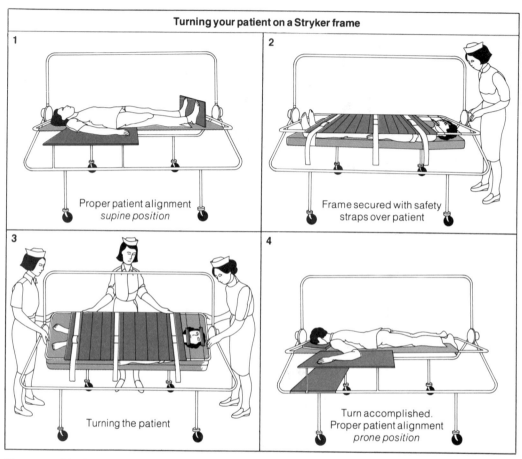

1 Proper patient alignment
supine position

2 Frame secured with safety
straps over patient

3 Turning the patient

4 Turn accomplished.
Proper patient alignment
prone position

Frames and beds
To care for a patient with spinal cord injuries who's immobilized on a frame or bed, you'll need to know the following: how to maintain proper spinal alignment; how to prevent further spinal cord damage; and how to promote healing of his bony injury. Additionally, you must take measures to prevent skin breakdown, and contracture deformities as explained in Chapter 3.

Stryker frame — A patient with severe neck or back injuries may be immobilized on a Stryker frame. Make sure you explain the purpose of the frame to your patient and his family; it will probably seem frightening to them. Unless your patient's prepared, he may fear falling when he's turned.

The Stryker frame uses an anterior and a posterior frame with canvas covers and thin padding over each. The frames, which are supported on a movable cart, have a pivot apparatus at each end. This allows you to change the patient's position to either prone or supine without altering his alignment.

To do this properly, follow the manufacturer's instructions or your hospital's procedure manual.

Further tips: Before turning your patient, secure any equipment he may have, such as I.V.s, Foley catheter, or respirator tubing to make sure it'll easily turn with him.

Some patients prefer to be turned more quickly than others. Place your patient's preference on his care plan along with the turning schedule.

• To prevent malalignment, check the equipment periodically and tighten the lacing of the canvases.

• To protect your patient's skin, place a foam mattress or padding on both frames and cover it with sheepskin.

• To aid in maintaining proper alignment, use a footboard, hand

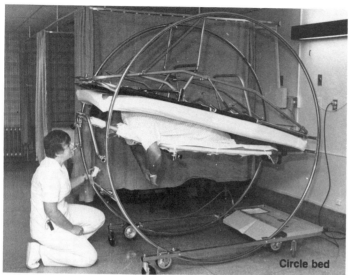

Circle bed

roll, bolsters and splints, as required.

• You may add arm rest wings to the frame at shoulder level. They'll permit your patient to rest his arms and will help maintain alignment.

• For meals, place him in prone position.

• For elimination, place him in supine position, with his bedpan under the opening in the canvas.

• When your patient's prone, carefully watch him for signs of respiratory problems. This position makes breathing more difficult.

• Help prevent your patient from feeling isolated, especially when he's prone. If he likes TV, place a set on the floor. Can he move his arms? He may wish to have books or hobbies on a tray under the frame.

• To care for a patient with skull tongs on a Stryker frame, always maintain traction, even when turning. During the turn, the nurse positioned at the patient's head will check pulley and weights.

Circle bed — You may be caring for a patient with neck or back

injuries who's immobilized in a Circle bed. This is a revolving bed with two major parts: a bottom mattress and a turning stretcher. A large, circular metal frame surrounds your patient, letting you turn him as often as necessary with minimal trauma or extraneous movement. To operate the bed electrically, you simply depress a push button. However, you can also operate it manually, if necessary.

As you can see in the photo above, your patient lies "sandwiched" between the bottom mattress and the turning stretcher, which you have secured over him. You change his position by turning him through an arc of the circle. *To minimize nausea and vertigo, don't interrupt the turn until he reaches the desired position.* For specific instructions on the turning procedure, consult the manufacturer's instructions or your hospital's procedure manual. *Nursing tips:*

• Familiarize patient and family with the Circle bed so they won't be frightened by it.

• Before turning your patient, make sure I.V. lines and other

equipment aren't tangled.

• Have another nurse help you turn your patient. One of you should operate the push button while the other watches the patient.

• If your patient has skull tongs, maintain traction during the turn. Make sure the equipment's secured to the mobile portion of the frame so it moves easily with him. Watch that the pulley clears the frame during the turn.

• For elimination, secure a bedpan to an opening on mattress or frame, depending on your patient's position.

• If the patient has copious respiratory drainage, provide a basin to collect secretions.

• When the patient's supine, give him prism glasses to increase his field of vision. With these, he can see all activity at eye level. If he can move his arms, he'll be able to read by holding a book normally, rather than overhead.

• To increase your patient's field of vision, attach a mirror to the upper part of the bed. Remember to remove it before turning him.

• In the prone position, a patient who has arm movement can take care of oral hygiene, write letters, play a game of solitaire, or read. Place the necessary materials on an overbed table within his reach.

Roto Rest bed — Suppose you're caring for a patient who's immobilized on a Roto Rest bed. Equipped with supportive packs and straps that keep the patient's body in proper alignment, this bed gently and continually rocks him in a cradle-like fashion. Besides alleviating the need for turning and positioning, the bed reduces the risk of fecal impaction and constipation because the continuous motion stimulates peristalsis. Be sure to consult the manufacturer's instructions as well as your hos-

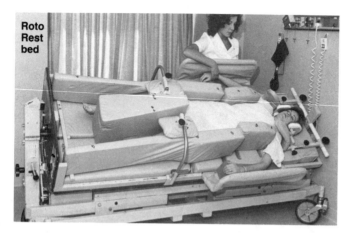

Roto Rest bed

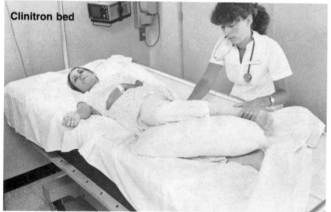

Clinitron bed

pital's procedure manual for specific operating information.
Nursing tips:
After bathing your patient, make sure soap residue is rinsed off his body and the support pack to prevent dermatitis.
• Before turning your patient, replace all packs and secure straps.
• For elimination, place bedpan under opening in bed.
• Routinely check the patient's knees for signs and symptoms of pressure.
• In case of power failure or motor malfunction, turn bed manually and lock.
• Because the bed's continuous motion promotes postural drainage, be prepared to suction patient frequently during his first 48 hours on the bed.
Clinitron bed — You may care for a patient who's immobilized on an air-fluidized support system like the one shown in the bottom photo on this page. A rectangular frame containing 1,600 pounds of silicone-coated glass beads (microspheres) covered with a closely woven monofilament polyester sheet makes up this special bed. The beads are fluidized by a flow of warm pressurized air, which floats the polyester cover. This bed provides a clean, controlled environment and reduces contact pressure.

Familiarize yourself with the manufacturer's instructions as well as your hospital's procedure when caring for a patient on this bed. In addition, here are some helpful guidelines:
• If a dressing's necessary, keep it as small as possible.
• If the patient has excessive wound drainage, place a porous dressing under his wound.
• If you use a petroleum-based or silver compound on the patient's skin, place an impervious covering over the filter sheet. This prevents these compounds from seeping into the microspheres.
• Be sure the system's cleaned every week to minimize the risk of contamination.
• For elimination, roll the patient away from you and push the bedpan into the microspheres. Reposition the patient on the bedpan. Afterward, defluidize the system and remove the bedpan by holding it flat as you roll the patient away from you with your other hand. Cleanse the patient, as usual. Fluidize the system and reposition the patient.
Regular hospital bed — If you're caring for your patient in a conventional hospital bed, you'll need a third person for all position changes. This third person coordinates the turn, standing at the head of the bed to guide the patient's head and the traction pulley. The other two people move the patient with a pull sheet to one side of the bed, then carefully log-roll him onto the desired side.

To prevent lateral flexion, place a small foam block under the patient's head while he's lying on his side.

Follow these guidelines — they'll help you minimize your patient's discomfort through the long and difficult period of immobilization.

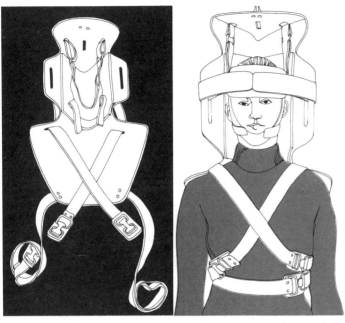

Safe transport
Moving an accident victim with possible spinal cord injury can be hazardous unless his head, neck, and thoracic spine are kept aligned. By providing constant cervical spine traction, the Meyer cervical orthosis allows health-care professionals to resuscitate, turn, and transport such a patient with less risk of further injury.

Now what can you do about it? First, try to understand the emotional stages your patient will go through to accept his injury. Though never distinct, these stages fall into these categories: initial shock, anger, depression, unrealistic hope for cure, and — finally — adaptation to disability.

Throughout all of them, or as many as you see while he's in your unit, your patient will need your psychologic support. Here are some stages you'll see:

• When your patient's going through the initial shock stage, expect him to use denial as a way to cope with his devastating injury. You may even see his family and some of the staff members going along with that denial. Don't be drawn into it, but don't push your patient into reacting differently before he's ready to. Answer all his questions truthfully. You won't hurt him doing this. He'll only hear what he wants to — and when he's ready.

• When your patient's going through the anger stage, expect the reality of his injury to hit him hard. He may lash out at anyone: you, his family, his doctor, God, and himself. Be understanding, but firm. Don't take his anger personally. Remember it's his behavior that's unacceptable, not the patient himself.

A passive exercise

Use passive range-of-motion exercises to help prevent contractures in your spinal-injured patient. For example, the exercise illustrated opposite is just one way to help prevent foot-drop. To do this properly, follow these instructions:

1. Hold the heel of your patient's foot with your hand so that your arm rests against the bottom of his foot. Place your other hand as shown in the picture.

2. Press your arm against the bottom of his foot to move the foot toward his leg. At the same time, pull on his heel as if you were trying to stretch his leg.

3. Move your arm back to the starting position.

4. Slide your hand up on the top of his foot below the toes. Push down on his foot to "point the toes." At the same time, push up against his heel. Return to the starting position and repeat.

Accomplished: Heel cord stretching.

Remember, you'll have to put each joint through a complete range of motion to prevent contractures. To plan an adequate exercise program for your spinal injured patient, check with the physical therapy department.

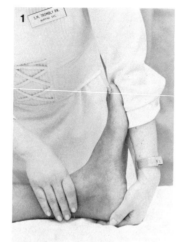
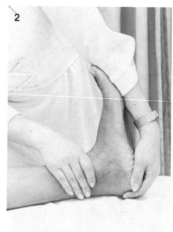
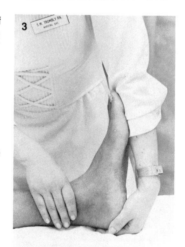
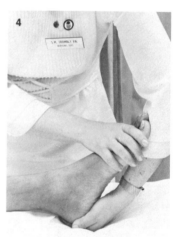

Remember the patient's family during this trying time, and explain what's happening to their loved one. Help them look on this period of verbal abuse as a temporary situation. If necessary, call in a psychiatric nurse clinician to consult with them and troubled staff members.

• When your patient's going through the depression stage, he may say he'd like to commit suicide. To him, the only thing worse than death is life as a quadriplegic. Encourage your patient to express his overwhelming feelings of despair and grief at this time.

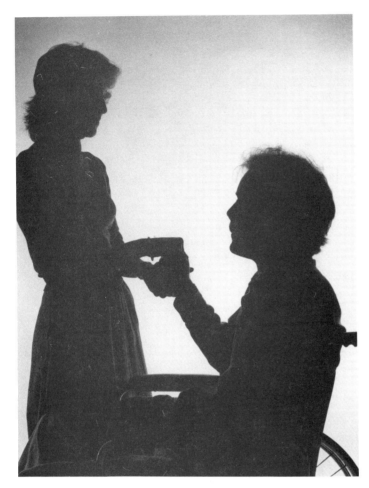

Sexuality and spinal cord injury

When a person becomes paralyzed, his sexual apprehensions are likely to start right away, not weeks or months after he's been transferred to a rehabilitation center. Because his feelings of self-worth and accomplishment are so closely tied to self-image and sexuality, anything that alters that image will mar his sense of personal fulfillment. Unless you acknowledge your patient's sexual anxiety quickly and attempt to deal with it, he may lose interest in all rehabilitation therapy. That's why your role in counseling's so important.

Obviously, you're not a psychologist. Nevertheless, you can talk to your patient as one human being to another and help him communicate his fears and hopes. Of course, to do this, you must first have come to terms with sexuality yourself. Answer all questions truthfully and calmly. If your patient confronts you with a question you can't answer, say you don't know but you'll find out.

To help your patient understand how his spinal injury will affect him sexually, be prepared to explain how his nervous system's been damaged and what level of sexual functioning he can expect. If you know the kind and extent of his injury, you can estimate how much physiological sexual capability remains.

For example, in complete cord injuries, loss of genital sensation occurs, although this doesn't necessarily mean loss of sexual pleasure. Most males with upper motor neuron injuries can have reflexogenic erections with cutaneous stimulation. Males with lower motor neuron injuries, however, will not have reflexogenic erections but may have psychogenic erections through erotic stimulation via sight, sound, smell, and touch. Male fertility is drastically reduced, since the nervous synchronization needed for ejaculation is disrupted.

Females with upper motor neuron lesions will have reflex clitoral engorgement and vaginal lubrication with local stimulation. Females with lower motor neuron lesions may need to use external lubrication.

Female fertility remains unchanged: A woman with spinal cord injuries can have normal pregnancies with vaginal deliveries. But a woman with an upper motor neuron disorder may experience dysreflexia during labor.

Both patient and partner will face difficult adjustments and may benefit from continued professional counseling. If they're encouraged to experiment, they'll probably attain a satisfactory sex life in time. Whatever activity the couple engages in must meet the approval of both partners. They must feel that sex, whatever form it takes for them, is natural and normal: an expression of themselves and their desire to share intimacy.

• When your patient's going through the stage where he unrealistically hopes for a cure, he may lose interest in his therapy program. If you're with him at this time, give him kindness and understanding, but don't let him regress. Perhaps a psychologist or social worker can help him gain a slow, gentle acceptance of reality.

• When your patient's finally accepted the seriousness of his injury, he'll probably settle down and adapt his life-style to his disability. He'll modify his former way of doing things and function as well as he can within the limits of his disability. Encourage this attitude by speaking positively and hopefully about his rehabilitation.

When he goes home

Besides the good physical care you'll give him, your patient needs help preparing for life outside the hospital. Try to provide that focus with the skills you've read about in this chapter. With the right care and a positive approach to new rehabilitation techniques, you'll give him a better chance to live a meaningful life.

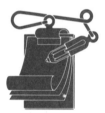

Remember these important points when caring for a patient with a spinal injury:
1. Suspect spinal cord injury in any patient with wounds of the face, neck, head, and shoulders, or in a patient who is unconscious from a head injury. Watch for paralysis of extremities, complaints of neck pain, and signs of spinal shock.
2. Immediately immobilize a patient with a suspected spinal injury. Take care not to move his neck or back.
3. Be aware that any spinal injury your patient experiences also affects your patient's autonomic nervous system. As a result, he may develop orthostatic hypotension, an inability to regulate his own body temperature, and neurogenic bladder and bowel.
4. Take care to prevent bladder distention, fecal impaction and decubitus ulcers. These complications may trigger autonomic dysreflexia.
5. Keep your patient positioned with pillows, Spenco boots, and hand and leg splints to prevent contractures.

SKILLCHECK

When his car went off the road, 17-year-old John Gaston suffered injuries that damaged his spinal cord completely at the T4 level.

1. When John arrives in the E.D., you observe that his blood pressure is 96/60 and his pulse is 60. Your understanding of spinal shock leads you to:
a) Place John in Trendelenburg position to combat shock.
b) Realize this is an expected response and anticipate an I.V. order.
c) Prepare to administer dopamine to reverse shock.
d) Realize these aren't signs of spinal shock and observe for hemorrhage.

2. Based on the level of John's cord damage, which of the following can you plan to include in his nursing care?
a) Physical and emotional care for a patient on a respirator.
b) An automatic bowel and bladder program.
c) Application and scheduling of splints to John's upper and lower extremities.
d) Daily wound care to John's tong site.

3. During a neurologic check on John's first night of hospitalization, you observe that his sensory loss is worsening. What do you do?
a) Mark it on his skin, and inform the doctor.
b) Apply icebags to the borderline areas where he's still feeling sensations.
c) Wait 24 hours until his condition stabilizes before you take further action.
d) Take no further action. His sensory losses are not significant.

4. Even after John's doctor has explained his injury to him, he says "I'm sure I'll be playing in next week's basketball game against Central High." How should you respond?
a) Tell John that his injury will prevent him from playing basketball.
b) Ask John to discuss this with his doctor.
c) Reassure John that miracles sometimes do happen; tell him not to give up hope.
d) Ignore John's remark, and change the subject.

5. How can you meet John's positioning and activity needs in the early phase of his hospitalization, if he's in a regular hospital bed?

a) With sufficient help, carefully assist John out of bed to a chair once a day.
b) Keep John in bed on his back with his head elevated to 90°.
c) Keep John flat in bed. Log-roll him from side to back to side at least once every 2 hours.
d) Alternate between supine and prone positions every 2 hours taking care to maintain alignment.

On her way to lunch, Jane Sylvester was struck on her head by a wrench which fell four stories from a repairman's scaffold. She was hospitalized with a subdural hemorrhage. Following aspiration of the clot, the surgeon inserted a subarachnoid screw to monitor her intracranial pressure.

6. How should you position Jane in bed?
a) Place her on her side and elevate her head to 30°, as ordered.
b) Place her in prone position and elevate her head, as ordered.
c) Keep her in supine position with her head lower than her body.
d) Place her on her side, but keep her flat.

7. Since Jane has a subarachnoid screw, what's an important nursing responsibility?
a) Maintain continuous irrigation of the screw.
b) Open the system every hour to allow drainage of excess cerebrospinal fluid.
c) Maintain a sterile system.
d) Inject the ordered dose of heparin into the system to prevent clotting.

8. Jane's latest arterial blood gases show that her PCO_2 has increased drastically. Her doctor orders mechanical hyperventilation. Why?
a) To prevent atelectasis and upper respiratory infection.
b) To lower arterial CO_2 which decreases blood volume, and therefore ICP.
c) To prevent respiratory depression due to hemorrhage of medulla.
d) To increase cerebral blood flow and improve oxygen supply to her brain.

(Answers on page 176)

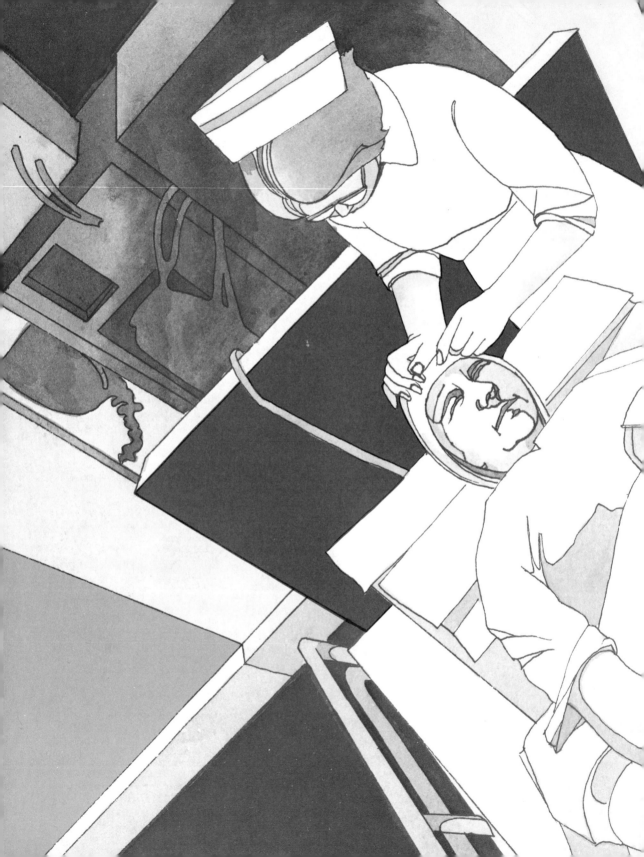

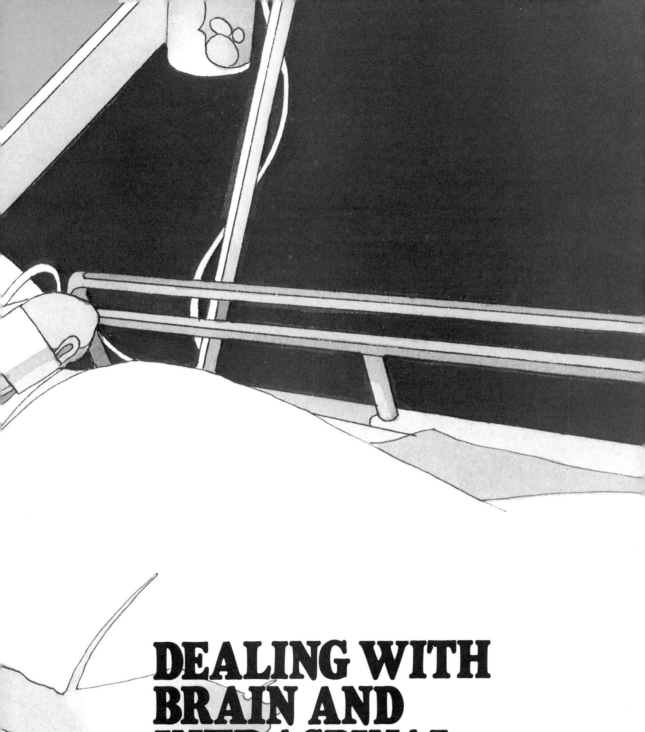

DEALING WITH BRAIN AND INTRASPINAL TUMORS

What complication commonly occurs in patients who have undergone a craniotomy?

If your patient has a supratentorial lesion, how may the doctor choose to surgically remove it?

What's the correct method for turning a patient who's recently had spinal surgery?

When is a spinal fusion necessary?

In a patient who's had spinal surgery, what signs and symptoms may signal spinal cord edema or permanent neurologic damage?

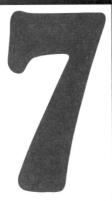

Intracranial Tumors
Giving expert pre- and postop care

BY CAROL L. MAYBERRY, RN, MS

"HE'S JUST NOT HIMSELF lately," Mrs. Stuber tells you outside your patient's room. "I knew it for sure when he started having trouble doing figures and had to quit his job...."

You're about to interview and assess her 60-year-old husband, who's been admitted to your unit. According to the admission form, his doctor wants him to have a complete neurologic checkup. "John acts so dragged out most of the time," Mrs. Stuber explains. "He's even started taking naps."

When you start assessing your patient's condition, you discover additional signs that warrant attention. For example, Mr. Stuber's gait shows left foot drop, and he says he sometimes has trouble buttoning his shirt and tying his shoes. Although he denies having visual difficulties, your optic check reveals vision loss in the left inferior quadrant. You document all these and other findings in detail, so you can incorporate them into your patient's care plan.

Does Mr. Stuber have a brain tumor?
What do Mr. Stuber's signs and symptoms suggest? Among other things, possible intracranial tumor (for a description of the various types, see page 129). Not all brain tumors cause the

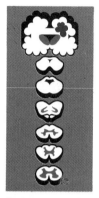

Pathophysiology
An intracranial tumor or *neoplasm* is an abnormal mass caused by excessive multiplication of cells within the cranium. The cause is unknown. As you know, tumors may be benign or malignant. Unlike tumors elsewhere, malignant brain tumors rarely metastasize outside the central nervous system.

Because there's no room for tissue growth within the brain, any intracranial tumor — benign or malignant — can be fatal. The patient may have local brain damage from the tumor; symptoms will depend on where it's located. Additionally, problems from increased intracranial pressure can occur.

same signs and symptoms, of course, because location and severity of lesions differ. Intracranial tumor may exist anytime a patient has frequent headaches, dizziness, seizures, visual impairment, speech difficulties, sensory loss, motor function loss, mental impairment, or personality changes. (However, there are other conditions that may cause these same symptoms.)

Do you know how to care for a patient with an intracranial tumor? When you assist him physically, can you recognize and plan for his needs? Suppose he needs surgery to remove a tumor? How do you prepare him for it? What special care will he require postoperatively? What about complications?

Obviously, I can't outline the exact nursing care needed by each patient with an intracranial tumor, because each patient — and tumor—is unique. But I can give you practical guidelines applicable to every case, as well as specific details relating to Mr. Stuber.

First things first
As I already explained, when Mr. Stuber enters the hospital, no one knows if he has a brain tumor. However, his initial assessment calls for these diagnostic tests: electroencephalogram (EEG), visual-field exam, computerized axial tomogram (CAT scan), skull X-ray, brain stem auditory-evoked potentials (BAEP), and visual-evoked responses (VER).

What do the above tests show in Mr. Stuber's case? Here are the results:
• EEG — shows right-sided dysrhythmia, indicating lesion in right hemisphere
• Visual-field exam — shows left inferior quadrant homonymous field defect (see page 57). Until the exam, Mr. Stuber had been ignorant of this defect because it didn't interfere with his daily activities.
• CAT scan — shows mass in right frontal and parietal lobes, with edema
• Skull X-ray — normal
• BAEP — shows waveform abnormalities from the right ear
• VER — shows waveform abnormalities.

Planning rehabilitation care early
Besides tests, Mr. Stuber gets the neurologic assessment explained in Chapter 2. Part of this determines his muscle

Intracranial tumors				
TUMOR TYPE	ORIGIN	GROWTH RATE	USUAL TREATMENT	PROGNOSIS
Glioma	Supportive or glial tissue			
The most common types of gliomas are the astrocytomas; malignant tumors composed of astrocytes, or star-shaped cells. Astrocytomas are usually graded in order of increasing malignancy (see below).				
— *Grade I or II astrocytoma*		Relatively slow	Complete surgical removal of as much as possible; after that, radiation. If location's inaccessible, surgery may not be possible.	Good Poor
— *Grade III or IV astrocytoma. (Sometimes called glioblastoma multiforme.)*		Rapid; highly invasive	Can't be completely removed by surgery; radiation only minimally effective. Current research involves chemotherapy.	Very poor
Meningioma	Meningeal tissue	Slow growing; usually encapsulated	Total surgical removal, if location's accessible; no radiation needed. If location's inaccessible, surgery may not be possible. Partial surgical removal· in certain cases (such as with increased vascularity); after that, radiation.	Very good Good, although tumors may recur in several years
Pituitary adenoma	Pituitary gland	Varies	X-ray therapy, radioactive implants, or cryosurgery. If other means fail to destroy all pituitary tissue, then surgical removal of pituitary gland.	Very good

Danger signals
In patients who've had intracranial surgery, any of these conditions may indicate a serious, perhaps life-threatening, situation:
- Onset of seizures
- Deteriorating level of consciousness
- Unilateral fixed dilated pupil
- Temperature above 101° F. (38.3° C.)
- Clear or excessive bloody drainage from wound
- Rebound hypertension if patient received nitroprusside sodium (Nipride) during surgery.

strength and tone, and helps you and the physical therapist plan care that'll prevent contractures and skin breakdown.

For example, soon after Mr. Stuber's admitted, you start using some of the rehabilitation measures described on pages 64 and 67. You and the therapist may alter this program later, if Mr. Stuber's condition changes.

What about surgery?
Should Mr. Stuber undergo surgery to remove his tumor? Before the doctor decides, he may need cerebral arteriogram to determine more about the lesion's location and vasculature.

How to prepare your patient for a cerebral arteriogram? Read the feature on diagnostic tests in the Appendices of this book. After the test, the patient needs care to minimize swelling and prevent bleeding.

Even though the doctor may not have determined Mr. Stuber's complete treatment plan, he will probably have these medications: dexamethasone (Decadron) 4 mg every 4 hours to reduce cerebral edema; and phenytoin (Dilantin) 300 mg daily to prevent seizures that may occur from a destructive lesion.

Discussing surgical risks
On page 131, you can read about surgical procedures used to remove intracranial tumors. In Mr. Stuber's case, the doctor recommends a craniotomy, which — like all procedures involving the brain and spinal cord — has special risks.

To illustrate: Suppose the surgeon has to remove or disturb normal brain tissue to get at Mr. Stuber's tumor. This could make his existing deficits worse and possibly add new ones.

Before Mr. Stuber can decide if he wants a craniotomy, he needs to know why the doctor recommends it and what complications may ensue. This will be a difficult decision for him to make, and he'll no doubt be worried. He may express fears about having a brain tumor, about losing his ability to function normally, and about dying.

Listen to his fears and encourage him to ask questions. Reinforce what the doctor's already told him; clear up any misunderstandings. Be informative and honest. Even though you can't guarantee a complete and uncomplicated recovery, you *can* instill confidence in his surgeon and the surgical procedure recommended.

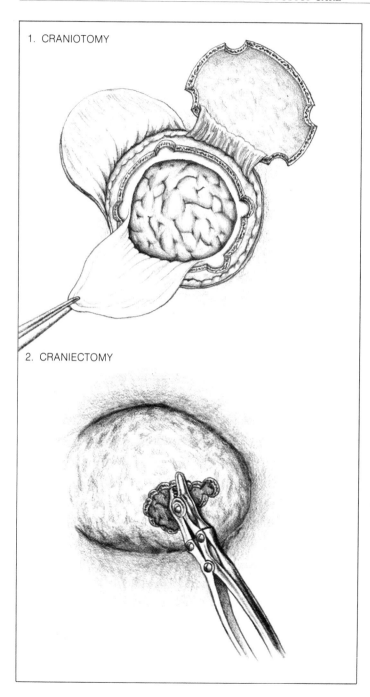

1. CRANIOTOMY

2. CRANIECTOMY

Surgery

CRANIOTOMY

The neurosurgeon makes a large opening in the cranium, forming a bone flap which remains attached to muscle tissue during the operation. Next, he incises the dura and opens it in the opposite direction (see illustration 1). Then he performs the needed surgery and finally sutures the flaps back in place.

The neurosurgeon commonly uses this procedure for supratentorial lesions. These, of course, are in the brain area above the tentorium.

CRANIECTOMY

The neurosurgeon removes a part of the patient's skull, varying in size from a small burr hole to a larger area. He uses a bone forceps to enlarge the original burr-hole opening when needed (see illustration 2). Then he performs the necessary brain surgery. He may freeze the bone and replace it later.

The neurosurgeon commonly uses this procedure for infratentorial lesions. These, of course, are in the area of the brain below the tentorium. However, he may use it for supratentorial lesions such as brain abscess, where there's a risk of bone infection. He may also use it if he anticipates intracranial expansion, such as from highly malignant tumors.

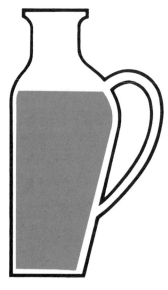

Diabetes insipidus
This disorder may occur after intracranial surgery. A patient's posterior pituitary gland temporarily stops secreting ADH (antidiuretic hormone). His renal tubules then fail to reabsorb enough water. When this happens, he'll complain of severe thirst and frequent urination. His urinary output can reach 10 liters or more a day. Its specific gravity may be as low as 1.001.

Watch for this problem, and report it at once; dehydration can occur rapidly. See that your patient gets the fluid and electrolyte replacement therapy the doctor orders.

Sometimes diabetes insipidus lasts only 2 or 3 days, before correcting itself. However, if problems continue or your patient loses too much fluid, the doctor may ask you to administer posterior pituitary extract.

On the next page, you'll find an explanation of another pituitary disorder.

Is he worried that he'll lose even more of his mental and physical capacities? Explain that *some* distressing symptoms may result from postop cerebral edema. When the edema eventually disappears, some of the symptoms may go with it. *However, don't mislead him. He may have residual effects.*

As you speak positively about the surgeon and the surgery, stress the benefits of your patient's ongoing therapy program. Reassure him and his wife that it'll continue — possibly with changes — after surgery.

Preparing Mr. Stuber

Mr. Stuber decides to undergo the recommended surgery. So outline the preop care he needs on his care plan and begin implementing it. Specifically, explain the procedures involved and what to expect afterwards.

For example, tell him that the surgeon will shave off some of his hair immediately before surgery (unless your orders say to do it earlier). Tell him that he'll awake with a large dressing — or bandage — on his head. Warn him that he may have a headache, as well as temporary swelling and discoloration around his eye on the affected side. However, reassure him that he'll receive medication to relieve pain.

Because Mr. Stuber will go to the ICU immediately after surgery, arrange a preop visit for him and his wife so they can see what it's like. Introduce them to the staff and explain some of the equipment. You'll probably find that the staff also benefits from this visit; they can see the patient's neurologic status firsthand and reinforce your teaching about postop procedures.

Consider postop needs

Now let's suppose your patient's undergone surgery and you're caring for him in the ICU. As I explained earlier, no two cases are exactly alike. For that reason, we won't discuss only the needs of Mr. Stuber, but those of all patients who've undergone this type of surgery.

Make sure you have a good care plan before you do anything. If it's properly written, it should include *specific* measures to prevent these complications: increased intracranial pressure, meningitis from wound infection, and respiratory difficulties.

Did your patient have a craniotomy or a craniectomy? Your

nursing orders must be tailored to his specific surgery, because postop care differs. You must also know whether his incision was supratentorial or infratentorial. I'll explain why when I tell you how to care for your patient.

Selecting the correct position

As soon as your patient returns from the O.R., place him on his side. If he had a craniectomy, make sure you don't place him on his operative side, because that'll put pressure directly on his brain (see page 131). *Never place him so his head's lower than the rest of his body.* As you read in earlier chapters, this may increase intracranial pressure.

Find out if your patient has a supratentorial or infratentorial incision. Then position him as follows, unless the doctor orders otherwise:

• Supratentorial — Elevate your patient's head 30° to increase venous return and help him breathe more easily. Turn him every 2 hours.

• Infratentorial — The doctor may ask you to keep your patient off his back for at least 48 hours. He may also want his head elevated 30°. Turn your patient every 2 hours, but make sure you have another nurse help you. Always use a turning sheet. Take care to support your patient's head and keep it aligned with his body.

No matter which position the doctor orders for your patient, document it on the care plan so everyone knows it. Tell the patient and his family and make sure they understand.

If all goes well, most patients will be ambulatory within 48 hours. Occasionally, a patient who's had an infratentorial incision will have to stay in bed longer.

Insuring good respiratory status

Observe your patient's respirations closely, noting the rate and pattern. Encourage him to deep-breathe and cough, but warn him not to do this strenuously. Listen to his breath sounds at least once every hour, and report any signs of respiratory distress *immediately*.

If the doctor orders suctioning, do it gently. In cases where suctioning doesn't help, the doctor may intubate him.

Make sure the patient's arterial blood gases are measured at regular intervals, and check the results. Remember, too high a level of carbon dioxide will produce cerebral vasodilation

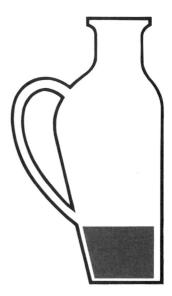

Inappropriate secretion of ADH
A disorder that's almost opposite to diabetes insipidus may also occur after your patient's had intracranial surgery. In this case, the posterior pituitary gland releases unneeded ADH. Renal tubules then reabsorb large amounts of water, but permit large amounts of sodium to be lost in the urine. As serum sodium continues to fall, your patient will lose his thirst mechanism and his appetite. His urinary output decreases, and its specific gravity increases. (More serious problems may include irritability, decreased level of consciousness, and muscular weakness.)

Recognize and report early symptoms. Make sure your patient restricts his fluids as his doctor orders, usually 500 to 1000 ml per day. With proper care, the problem usually corrects itself.

Hair and scalp care

After your patient's had intracranial surgery, the doctor may want you to apply antiseptic to the site to help prevent infection. You may also apply antibacterial ointment to keep the skin supple around the suture line.

Once the doctor's removed the sutures — usually 7 to 10 days after the operation — thoroughly wash the patient's scalp and hair.

Like many patients, he may be concerned about his physical appearance while his hair's growing in. Suggest he wear a wig or cap, such as an O.R. cap. A female patient may choose to wear a wig or turban.

Because treated skin's more susceptible to sunburn, any patient receiving radiation treatments should wear a head covering when outdoors.

which increases cerebral edema. Notify the doctor.

Monitoring fluid and electrolyte balance

When your patient arrives in the ICU, he'll be getting I.V. fluids and have a Foley catheter in place. Chances are his fluid intake will be greatly restricted to minimize temporary cerebral edema and prevent increased intracranial pressure. Keeping this danger in mind, *make sure I.V. fluids don't infuse too rapidly*.

Monitor intake and output, and document your findings carefully on a flow sheet. Always report urinary output that falls as low as 20 ml per hour for 2 consecutive hours. Record urinary specific gravity every 2 hours. Weigh your patient, according to doctor's orders.

Keep a close watch on the patient's electrolyte levels. Remember, decreased sodium and chloride levels may produce weakness, lethargy, and coma. Low potassium levels may cause confusion and lack of responsiveness.

Caution: For the patient who's undergone intracranial surery, a fluid and electrolyte imbalance warrants treatment. He runs a risk of developing seizures.

After a while, the doctor will probably order oral fluids for your patient. Before you give them, check your patient's gag reflex. This is particularly important if he's had an infratentorial incision, because the surgery may have affected his glossopharyngeal and vagus nerves.

If your patient vomits after he's started oral fluids, discontinue them and notify the doctor. He may want you to restart I.V. therapy. Vomiting can increase intracranial pressure.

Checking the patient's dressing

Chances are you won't be expected to change the patient's dressing. But you'll have to check it at least once an hour while he's in the ICU and report any abnormal findings.

Most patients will return from the O.R. with a closed drainage system, such as Neurovac. Note the amount, color, and odor of drainage and document it. Normally, you'll see some serosanguineous drainage at first, but if bleeding's excessive, call the doctor immediately. Notify him at once if the drainage is clear or yellow; that may indicate a cerebrospinal fluid leak.

As I mentioned earlier, your patient runs the risk of meningitis if he develops a wound infection. Note any color or odor when you check drainage. Report signs of infection immediately.

Get a doctor at once if you notice dressing tightness. That may indicate swelling — a sign of increased intracranial pressure. Remember, such swelling can occur any time during healing. Don't stop watching your patient for this danger sign after his dressing's been removed.

Continue ongoing neurologic checks

Obviously, you'll continue to assess your patient's neurologic status and vital signs as explained in Chapter 2. Do this at least once every half hour until he's stable, unless the doctor orders more frequent checks. Later, check your patient once every 2 hours. Document all findings.

Call the doctor promptly if you see signs of increased intracranial pressure (see page 92), cerebrospinal fluid leak, infection, or respiratory distress. If the patient has a seizure, care for him as described in Chapter 9 and document your observations. Report a seizure to the doctor immediately.

Provide supportive care

What else will your patient need while he's in the ICU? Along with everything else, the doctor will probably want you to:

• Ensure a quiet, calm environment for your patient. Warn him not to pull at his dressing, and possibly enlist his family's help to keep him from becoming restless. If these measures fail, the doctor may order mitten restraints. Don't use more confining restraints; they may upset your patient further. Remember, agitation can increase intracranial pressure.

• Maintain seizure precautions, as outlined in Chapter 9.

• Provide eye care. Apply ice to swollen lids. Lubricate lids and area around eye, as per doctor's orders.

• Continue range-of-motion exercises, as planned for in the patient's ongoing physical therapy program.

• Give necessary medications (see this page).

• Keep the family well informed about the patient's condition, and offer reassurance and emotional support.

What happened to Mr. Stuber?

As you probably recall, Mr. Stuber underwent a craniotomy. The surgeon partially removed a low-grade astrocytoma.

While he was still in the ICU, the doctor recommended

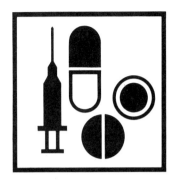

Medications
After your patient's had intracranial surgery, the doctor may ask you to give him these medications:
• Steroids, to prevent cerebral edema
• Anticonvulsants, to prevent seizures
• Stool softeners, to prevent increased intracranial pressure from straining
• Mild analgesics, to control pain.

**Computerized axial tomography
(CAT scan)**
If the doctor suspects your patient
has a brain tumor, he'll probably
order computerized axial
tomography (CAT scan). To learn
how to prepare your patient for this
test and care for him afterwards,
see the Appendices.

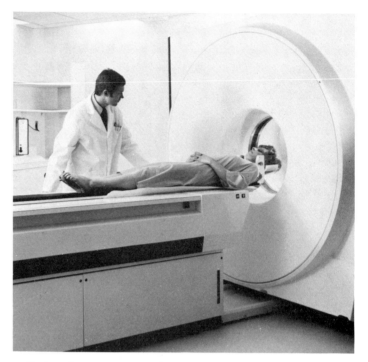

radiation therapy as part of Mr. Stuber's continuing treatment
plan. As Mr. Stuber's nurse, you reinforced the doctor's explanation by answering questions about radiation therapy.
You told Mr. Stuber what to expect and how to care for his
scalp while he's receiving therapy.

Mr. Stuber continued taking the anticonvulsant drugs and
steroids he received in the hospital, although the steroid dosage was reduced gradually. Because he still runs the risk of
cerebral edema, he'll keep on taking steroids throughout radiation therapy.

The risk of hydrocephalus
Fortunately, Mr. Stuber had an uncomplicated recovery. Not
every patient is so lucky. Some develop hydrocephalus, an
abnormal accumulation of cerebrospinal fluid within the cranial cavity. As we already explained in Chapter 5, such accumulation increases intracranial pressure.

If the doctor suspects hydrocephalus, he'll probably order a
computerized axial tomogram (CAT scan). This test is the
most reliable indication of ventricular enlargement.

VENTRICULOPERITONEAL SHUNT

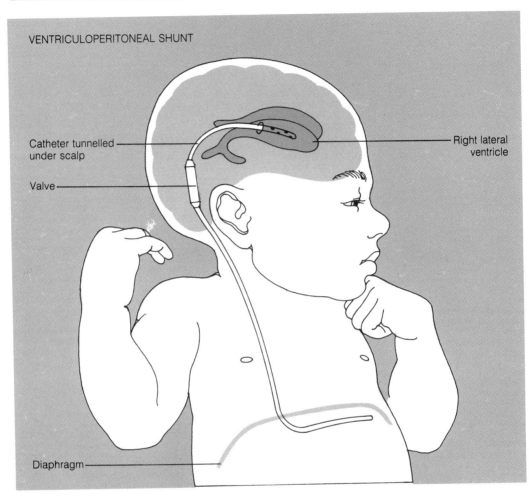

Catheter tunnelled under scalp

Valve

Diaphragm

Right lateral ventricle

Treating hydrocephalus
The most common surgical treatment for hydrocephalus is the ventriculoperitoneal shunt, although you may see a patient with a ventriculoatrial shunt. For the ventriculoperitoneal shunt, the doctor inserts a catheter into the patient's ventricular system, usually via a lateral ventricle. Then he attaches it to another catheter, which he tunnels through the subcutaneous tissue to a point below the diaphragm, where he can puncture the

peritoneal sac. Between these catheters he places a valve system and inserts it under the patient's scalp, behind his ear.

Pre- and postop care of a shunt patient is the same as for a craniotomy patient (see page 132).

After the shunt's in place, an infant may be irritable. An older child may get headaches when he tries to sit up. Help him to sit up by gradually raising his head in stages, about 20° at a time. Reassure him that his headaches will stop when he's

accustomed to the shunt.

Before discharge, give the patient's family clear instructions about his shunt. Tell them to report at once any symptoms of increased ICP, such as restlessness, headaches, or decreased level of consciousness. These may indicate that the shunt is blocked.

They should also call the doctor immediately if signs of infection occur: increased temperature, headaches, or nuchal rigidity.

To relieve the pressure of hydrocephalus, the doctor may try surgery. For example, he may:

• remove the obstruction blocking the normal flow of cerebrospinal fluid in the ventricles

• install a shunt by placing a catheter within the ventricle to route the cerebrospinal fluid around the obstruction to an area where it can be reabsorbed in the circulatory system and eventually excreted. To learn about ventricular shunts and how to care for the patient who has one, read page 137.

The triple challenge
By the time Mr. Stuber was ready for discharge, he no longer had all of the symptoms he came in with. His physical condition and mental outlook improved daily, though he still had to return as an outpatient for radiation therapy.

Good nursing care had a lot to do with Mr. Stuber's excellent recovery. Can you give it? In this chapter, I've outlined how you can help the patient with an intracranial tumor. His nursing care presents a triple challenge: You must know how to do an ongoing neurologic assessment, provide complete pre- and postop care, and assist with rehabilitative therapy.

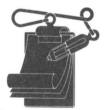

Remember these important points when caring for a patient with an intracranial tumor:
1. Carefully explain all diagnostic tests, including the CAT scan, visual-field exam, EEG, skull X-ray, BAEP, and VER.
2. After intracranial surgery, consider these conditions life-threatening: onset of seizures, deteriorating level of consciousness, unilateral fixed dilated pupil, temperature above 101°F. (30.3°C.), clear or excessive bloody wound drainage, and rebound hypertension (if nitroprusside sodium was administered during surgery).
3. Check to be sure I.V. fluids aren't infusing too rapidly. Remember, after surgery your patient's fluid intake probably will be restricted to minimize temporary cerebral edema and prevent increased intracranial pressure.
4. Notify the doctor if your patient's dressing appears tight or if you observe any sign of infection.
5. Be aware that insertion of a ventriculoperitoneal shunt is the most common treatment for hydrocephalus.

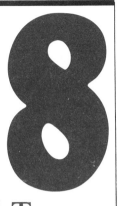

Intraspinal Tumors
Meeting your patient's surgical needs

BY NORMA M. ISAACS, RN, BN

AS 14-YEAR-OLD Ben Cooley sits anxiously on the edge of his bed, his mother talks rapidly. "I don't know why he didn't tell me he was having problems," she blurts out. "You can't imagine how scared I got when I saw him at breakfast a couple mornings ago."

Because her job as a real estate agent kept her away from home a lot, Ben's mother rarely spent time with him. She hadn't noticed his rapidly progressing muscle weakness until that morning. Then it was obvious: He couldn't even pick up his glass.

According to Ben's medical history, his symptoms began 6 months earlier when he complained of a stiff neck. His mother didn't take him to a doctor because it didn't seem serious. Ben never mentioned it again, though the pain and stiffness persisted.

Within 2 months, Ben — a promising school athlete — noticed other signs that distressed him. For example, he could no longer play soccer because he had trouble running, kicking the ball, and maintaining his balance. He gave up tennis because he couldn't grasp the racquet securely. His neck pain and stiffness grew worse, progressing down his arms.

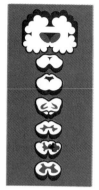

Pathophysiology
What is an intraspinal tumor? Any abnormal mass from excessive multiplication of cells encroaching on the bony spinal canal. These are classified according to their relationship to dura and cord, as well as by histological type (see page 141). As you know, a tumor may be benign or malignant. Many times it's a metastatic lesion arising from a primary site located elsewhere in the body. Both benign and malignant tumors can cause upper and lower motor neuron disturbances, as well as sensory deficits.

Today, Ben's a patient in your unit. When you see him, his condition has deteriorated so much that he can no longer stand or walk without help. Fortunately, he can still breathe adequately and has normal bowel and bladder function. He's obviously frightened, so you try to reassure him.

What does all this suggest? Ben's symptoms point to spinal cord involvement. He may have an intraspinal tumor, but the doctor can't tell without certain diagnostic tests. Following a clinical examination, the doctor will probably order the following, along with routine lab tests and X-rays, to determine any existing metastases:

• lumbar puncture. This may show a decrease in cerebrospinal fluid (CSF) pressure, which indicates a subarachnoid block (often found in patients with intraspinal tumors). CSF analysis will show an elevation in total proteins.

• spinal X-ray. This may show destruction of bone or a space-occupying lesion, which will indicate the area of involvement.

• computerized axial tomogram (CAT scan) of spine. This may help pinpoint the location of an intraspinal tumor.

• myelography. This may demonstrate the presence of a tumor.

Naturally, you'll prepare Ben and his family for these tests by explaining what they are and why they are necessary. Then give him the physical care he needs before and after each test. (For further details about diagnostic tests and the nursing care involved, see the Appendices.)

What type of tumor?
Diagnostic tests indicate that Ben probably has an intraspinal tumor in the upper cervical area. However, tests alone can't identify the exact type of tumor (see page opposite.) For this the doctor will need a biopsy.

Nevertheless, a patient's history, and signs and symptoms can provide the doctor with valuable clues about the tumor. For example, suppose your patient has an extramedullary tumor. Chances are he'll first complain of pain in the area where the tumor compresses nerve roots. Then as his tumor grows, he'll gradually develop other problems: sensory loss, weakness, and muscle atrophy.

However, suppose your patient has an intramedullary tumor, which will interfere first with nerve-impulse transmis-

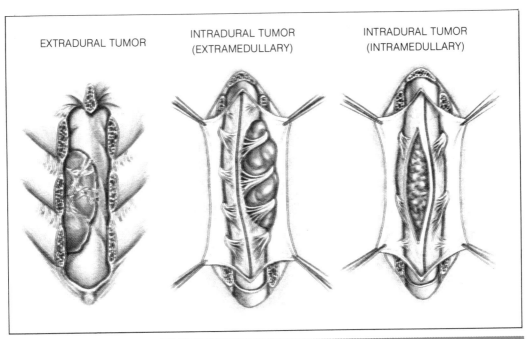

EXTRADURAL TUMOR   INTRADURAL TUMOR (EXTRAMEDULLARY)   INTRADURAL TUMOR (INTRAMEDULLARY)

Intraspinal tumors

Classification — *Intraspinal tumors may be classified by location in reference to the dura.*

TYPE	INCIDENCE	TREATMENT	PROGNOSIS
Extradural	25% to 50% of all intraspinal tumors Mostly malignant metastatic lesions	Relieve cord compression by surgical laminectomy, radiation, chemotherapy, or combinations.	Poor
Intradural	50% to 75% of all intraspinal tumors	See below.	See below.
— Extramedullary	Most frequent Mostly benign meningiomas and neurofibromas	Complete surgical removal of most is possible. If not, partial removal followed by radiation.	Usually very good if cord's not damaged by compression.
— Intramedullary (within cord)	Least frequent Mostly malignant gliomas	Many can't be completely removed surgically. Radiation therapy shows only some temporary improvement.	Very poor

sion within the spinal cord. In this case, pain probably won't be a problem until later. Chances are he'll complain first of a gradual loss of cutaneous and proprioceptive sensations below the lesion's level. This occurs as the tumor affects sensory tracts.

Then, as the tumor grows and affects spinal cord motor tracts, the patient will develop spastic motor weakness, which will lead to complete paralysis. Rapidly developing paralysis may also indicate an extradural tumor. To review how spinal-cord lesions can disrupt motor and sensory functions to this degree, read Chapter 6.

Preparing Ben for surgery

As I said earlier, the doctor thinks Ben's neurologic problems stem from an intraspinal tumor in his upper cervical area. Obviously he can't tell whether or not he can remove the tumor until he performs the recommended surgery (see opposite page). At that time, he'll also do a biopsy to see if the tumor's malignant.

How will you prepare Ben and his family for spinal surgery? During the period before it, the doctor will probably want you to do the following:

• Continue assessing Ben's neurologic status. Be alert for signs of deterioration: for example, further sensory or motor function loss, incontinence, or a combination of these. If any of these occur, notify the doctor promptly. He may want to perform surgery immediately, to prevent further neurologic deficits or worsening of existing deficits.

Anytime you do a neurologic assessment, document your findings and update your patient's care plan, if necessary. Is his condition changing? His care plan will probably need changing, also.

• Watch vital signs closely. Any lesion located in the upper cervical area may affect muscles needed for respirations. Call the doctor immediately if you notice signs of respiratory distress. Do all you can to prevent respiratory problems by caring for your patient as outlined in Chapter 6.

• Provide good skin care to prevent skin breakdown. (For tips on this, see Chapter 3.)

• Urge your patient to use whatever ability he has left, thus minimizing the chance of contractures. For example, can he get out of bed? Brush his teeth? Feed himself? Encourage him.

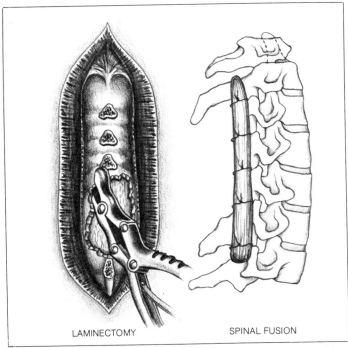

LAMINECTOMY   SPINAL FUSION

Suppose your patient can't complete an entire task by himself. Urge him to do what he can, and praise him for his efforts. In Ben's case, he can roll independently from right to left, but not back again. He also needs help standing and getting from his bed to the chair.

You may want to start some passive range-of-motion exercises before surgery (see Chapter 3). Doing so will introduce your patient to the rehabilitative physiotherapy he'll need postoperatively.

• Give adequate psychologic support. Your patient and his family will naturally be quite upset by the doctor's tentative diagnosis and the prospect of surgery. Listen to their fears and reassure them all you can. Obviously, you can't guarantee that everything will be all right. But you can make things easier by explaining what will happen before and after surgery.

• Meet nutrititional needs. Consult with the dietitian to make sure your patient has the high-calorie, high-protein diet the doctor's probably ordered. If your patient's rundown or anemic, he'll lack the resistance he needs to ward off possible postop infection.

Spinal surgery

LAMINECTOMY
In this procedure, the surgeon makes an incision over the involved vertebral area and extends it down through fascia and muscles to the laminae (flattened parts on sides of vertebral arch). Then he removes one or more laminae or portions of them.

Surgeons perform a laminectomy to reach dura, disc, or cord, and complete needed surgery in those areas.
Postop nursing care:
• Your patient may get out of bed within 24 hours after surgery, although this isn't always so.
• Check for: hemorrhage; motor or sensory deficits; loss of bowel or bladder functioning.
• Position as ordered; maintain alignment; log-roll when turning.

SPINAL FUSION
Occasionally, after laminectomy, the patient needs spinal fusion. For example, this may be needed if a lesion or injury has caused an unstable spine. To accomplish spinal fusion, the surgeon will remove bone from part of the patient's body (usually the iliac crest) and graft it onto the vertebrae.
Postop nursing care:
• Prepare patient for possible extended bedrest in flat position. Tell him he'll have to wear a back brace when he gets out of bed.
• Prevent movement at fusion site. Position the patient as ordered, maintain alignment, and log-roll when turning.
• Check for hemorrhage; motor or sensory deficits; and loss of bowel or bladder functioning. Occasionally, a surgeon inserts Harrington rods after spinal fusion. These act as temporary internal splints to help the bones unite properly.

Herniated intervertebral disc

As you know, an intervertebral disc, which acts as a shock absorber, is located between the vertebral bodies. Two layers of cartilage separated by a gelantinous center, or nucleus pulposus, make up each disc. A protective fibrous tissue ring known as the annulus fibrosus surrounds both layers and extends to anterior, posterior, and longitudinal ligaments, as well as vertebral bodies.

An injury can tear the annulus fibrosus, permitting part of the nucleus pulposus to herniate through the posterior ligament into the spinal canal. This is called a ruptured, herniated, or "slipped" disc. Most herniated discs occur in the lumbar and lumbosacral regions. Pressure on nerve roots in those areas cause:
 • severe low back pain and spasm made worse by sneezing, coughing, and bending
 • muscular weakness in affected leg
 • radiating sciatic pain to leg and foot
 • sensory changes in the involved dermatome.

Initial treatment is usually conservative. The doctor may want the patient to have bedrest, (usually in pelvic traction) and physical therapy (heat and exercises). Medications may include muscle relaxants and analgesics during the acute period.

If this treatment fails, the doctor may perform a laminectomy or a hemilaminectomy to remove the protruding nucleus pulposus. Sometimes surgery will include spinal fusion. Important: If your patient has a ruptured *cervical* intervertebral disc, he'll probably complain of arm pain and weakness.

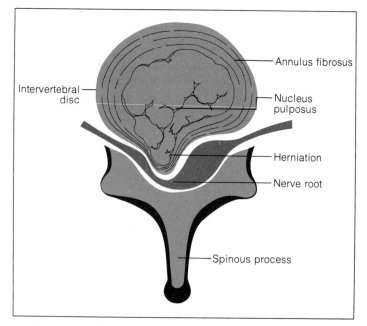

 • Complete all nursing measures needed to prepare your patient for the O.R. For example, see that a Foley catheter's inserted, unless the doctor orders intermittent catheterization. Tell your patient what to expect when he wakes up from anesthesia. Explain that he'll receive medication for pain. Show him the log-rolling procedure you'll use to turn him regularly after surgery, and stress the importance of proper positioning, deep-breathing, and coughing.

Ben's surgery

What does Ben's surgery reveal? During a decompressive laminectomy and exploration of the cord in Ben's upper cervical area, the surgeon discovers an extensive — and inoperable — tumor. Pathology reports indicate that it's a high-grade astrocytoma of the spinal cord.

Though you're aware that Ben's prognosis is poor, you also know the doctor will plan treatment to help him. For example, Ben will continue a rehabilitative therapy program to lessen existing neurologic deficits and minimize the progression of new ones. After discharge from the hospital, he'll also receive radiation therapy. Together, these treatment plans will provide Ben and his family with some hope for the future. You can do your part to encourage that hope with a positive outlook, adequate teaching, and reassurance.

Meeting postoperative needs
No matter what type of surgery or intraspinal tumor your patient has, you must individualize his postop care to meet his needs. Like other patients, Ben will have special needs that you'll include in his care plan. His family will also need considerable emotional support, because Ben's tumor is inoperable.

However, certain guidelines apply to all patients after surgery for any intraspinal tumor. So let's consider these for the rest of this chapter. When your patient returns from the O.R., the doctor will probably want you to pay attention to the following:

• Positioning and activity. Find out exactly how the doctor wants your patient positioned. In some cases, he may want the patient to lie on his back immediately after surgery. In other cases, he may want the patient to lie on his side. No matter what position your patient's in, make sure his back is properly aligned and pressure areas receive attention.

Chances are, the doctor will not want you to elevate your patient's head at first. Check his orders carefully and make sure the information is recorded on the care plan. As an extra precaution, post a notice about it on the bed.

Don't give your patient a pillow until you check the doctor's orders. He may not want him to have one if surgery involved the cervical area. Instead, he may order a soft cervical collar to keep the patient from turning his head to either side or flexing it forward.

Wait for the doctor to tell you when he wants the patient turned for the first time postop. Then get an assistant to help you and turn your patient, using the log-roll method. Do this once every 2 hours, as illustrated on page 146. Make sure you document it.

Nursing tip: If your patient's position changes so you have to move him back toward the head of the bed, use a turning sheet but, first, make sure you get someone to help you. Never lift by supporting him under the shoulders or armpits. You could do serious damage if he had cervical or thoracic surgery.

Turning your patient regularly will help prevent contractures and skin breakdown. In addition, you'll want to start the passive range-of-motion exercises outlined by the physical

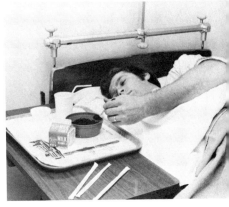

Side order
After extensive spinal surgery, your patient will have to eat lying on his side until he can sit in a straight chair for his meals. Place his tray close to his bed so he can reach it easily. Make sure he has enough drinking straws. And allow him plenty of time to finish.

Log-rolling

Here's the correct way to turn your patient who's had spinal surgery: To do this, you'll need two or three nurses, depending on the patient's size. Before moving him, lower the side rails of his bed, place a pillow between his legs, and have him cross his arms on his chest. Be sure the bed is flat.

1. With you and your helper on the same side of the bed, extend your arms under the patient's shoulders, back, buttocks, and legs. Then pull him over to the side of the bed. Alternatively, you may use a pull sheet.

2. Have your helper move to the other side of the bed. Together, roll the patient onto his side. Don't allow him to twist his back; roll his entire body all at once. While the patient's on his side, straighten the bed linen.

3. With the patient on his side, prop a pillow against his back for support and leave the pillow between his legs.

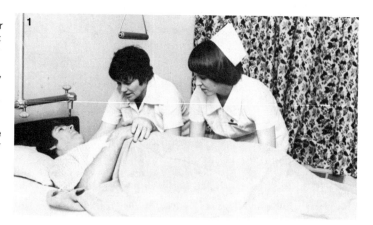

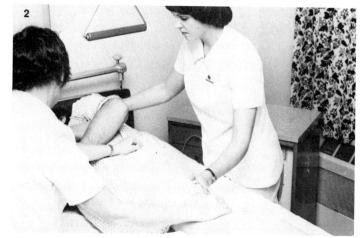

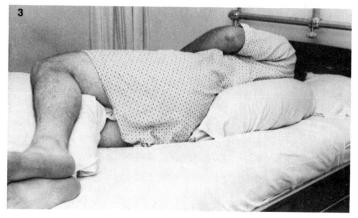

therapy department. Later on, you can encourage more active exercises as your patient's condition improves.

• Continue assessing your patient's neurologic status as you did preoperatively. To do this accurately, keep a dermatome chart at the bedside and refer to it (see page 42). Document your findings and report changes to the doctor. Your observations will help him determine if the surgery was successful or if it caused further damage.

Be especially alert for signs of deterioration. Sudden incontinence or continuing loss of motor or sensory function may indicate spinal-cord edema or permanent neurologic damage.

• Check vital signs. Call the doctor immediately if your findings suggest infection or hemorrhage (see the danger signs on this page). However, don't be alarmed if your patient's temperature elevates to 100° F. (37.8° C.). This is probably from meningeal irritation during surgery.

• Maintain adequate respirations. Encourage your patient to cough and deep-breathe, as you instructed him before surgery. Turn him regularly, according to the guidelines already mentioned.

Call the doctor at once if you notice respiratory distress, which may occur from temporary spinal-cord edema. This constitutes a particular risk for patients after cervical surgery.

• Check wound dressings. Do this at least once every 2 hours, when you turn your patient, or as ordered. Expect some bloody or serosanguineous drainage if the doctor inserted drains during surgery.

Are the dressings saturated? This suggests a possible wound rupture, which — if left untreated — can lead to infection. Don't try to remove them. Just reinforce them with sterile dressings and call the doctor at once.

• Monitor your patient's intake and output, and maintain proper fluid and electrolyte balance. Chances are, your patient will receive I.V. fluids for at least 24 hours after surgery. He may also return from the O.R. with a Foley catheter in place, unless the doctor's ordered intermittent catheterization. Infuse fluids exactly as ordered and monitor intake and output carefully.

Nursing tip: Can your patient use a bedpan? Never lift him on the pan while he's lying on his back; such a move could put pressure on his operative site. Instead, carefully log-roll him to his side.

Danger signals
Any of these conditions in patients with intraspinal tumors may indicate a serious, perhaps life-threatening, situation:
• Appearance of new sensory or motor deficits, or worsening of existing ones
• Saturated bloody dressing
• Difficult breathing (especially after cervical surgery).

Then place the bedpan in position and gently turn him back onto it.

• Ensure adequate nutrition. Within a day or so your patient will probably resume oral feedings. Don't let anyone elevate his head for this, however. Keep him on his side and place the tray next to him on the bed (see the illustration on page 145).

Document these instructions on his care plan. Make sure his family understands, and post a notice on his bed.

• Keep your patient as comfortable as possible. After spinal surgery, he'll no doubt have severe pain. To relieve it, the doctor will probably order narcotics to be given I.M., though not morphine, which can depress respirations.

Consider future treatment plans

As I said earlier, each patient's case is different. Your nursing orders will vary from patient to patient, depending on the outcome of surgery and the degree of neurologic damage. For many patients the future may be brighter than it once was. Improved radiation, chemotherapy, and rehabilitative therapy have improved the prognosis for intraspinal tumors. And don't forget, surgery can be successful if a tumor's detected early enough.

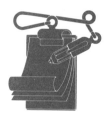

Remember these important points when caring for a patient with an intraspinal tumor:

1. Minimize the risk of contractures by encouraging your patient to do as much as possible for himself.

2. Following surgery, be sure your patient is properly aligned and any pressure areas are properly supported.

3. Consider any of the following conditions a serious life-threatening situation: appearance of new sensory or motor deficits, or worsening of existing ones; saturated bloody dressing; and breathing difficulties.

4. Be aware of the signs and symptoms of a herniated intervertebral disc: severe low back pain and spasm made worse by sneezing, coughing, and bending; muscular weakness in affected leg; sciatic pain radiating to leg and foot; and sensory changes in the involved dermatome.

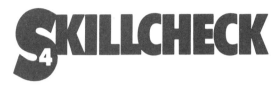

SKILLCHECK

You're caring for Jim Nesbitt who's just had a lumbar spinal fusion. His doctor wrote strict orders to prevent trauma at the fusion site.

1. How should you position Mr. Nesbitt when he returns from surgery?
a) Position him flat, maintaining spinal alignment.
b) Elevate his head 30° to prevent increased intracranial pressure.
c) Elevate his legs 45° to 60° to prevent pressure on the spinal canal.
d) Have him lie prone to prevent wound disruption.

2. The doctor gives permission for Mr. Nesbitt to be turned for the first time. How do you do this?
a) Instruct your patient to lift himself carefully to the side of the bed with a trapeze. Then help him to turn on his side.
b) Follow turning instructions for Stryker frame or CircOlectric bed because he can't be cared for in a regular bed.
c) Instruct him to remain rigid. Then, with assistance turn him as a unit using a pull sheet.
d) With assistance, flex your patient's legs slightly, and bend his head gently forward. Then use a pull sheet to turn him to his side.

3. Your care of Mr. Nesbitt is easier because you prepared him well for his surgery. Which of the following did you tell him preoperatively?
a) That he wouldn't be ambulatory for at least 5 months.
b) That he'd probably have to wear a back brace for a while after his surgery.
c) That, for a time at least, he'd definitely have metal rods inserted in his back.
d) That he'd have to use a cane for support for the rest of his life.

4. How should you position Mr. Nesbitt for meals in the early postoperative period?
a) Elevate his head 45° to prevent aspiration.
b) If ordered, turn him on his side but keep him flat.
c) If ordered, keep him prone with his tray below him.
d) Keep him supine, but turn his head to the side.

5. Following Mr. Nesbitt's surgery, which of these assessment checks is most important?
a) Pupillary checks
b) Coordination checks
c) Sensory checks
d) Checks for increased ICP.

You're taking care of 50-year-old Martha Hedges in ICU. This morning she had a craniotomy and the neurosurgeon removed a low-grade glioma from her left posterior frontal lobe.

6. How should you position Mrs. Hedges' head?
a) Flat to maintain optimal alignment.
b) Elevated 30° to prevent an increase in ICP.
c) Lower than the rest of her body to increase blood supply to the operative site.
d) Elevated 90° to promote venous return.

7. You notice while checking Mrs. Hedges dressing that it's getting very tight. What should you do?
a) Report it to the doctor at once.
b) Nothing. This is an expected response from surgery.
c) Remove the dressing until the doctor comes.
d) Loosen the dressing and re-check in 30 minutes.

8. Which of Mrs. Hedges' assessment findings warrants immediate action?
a) You observe serosanguineous drainage on her dressing.
b) Her temperature increases to 99.5° F. (37.5° C.).
c) Her left pupil remains dilated.
d) Her PCO_2 has dropped slightly from the last normal blood-gas result.

9. Several days later, Mrs. Hedges asks you when she can have her "terrible head dressing" removed and wear her new blond wig. How do you reply?
a) "It won't be possible to wear your wig until your radiation treatments are completed."
b) "In a few days your doctor will probably remove your sutures. Then you can leave your dressing off and wear your wig."
c) "Ask your doctor. He will probably want you to wear a soft scarf for awhile."
d) "Wigs are irritating to your scalp. You may wear one but wear your dressing under it."

(Answers on page 176)

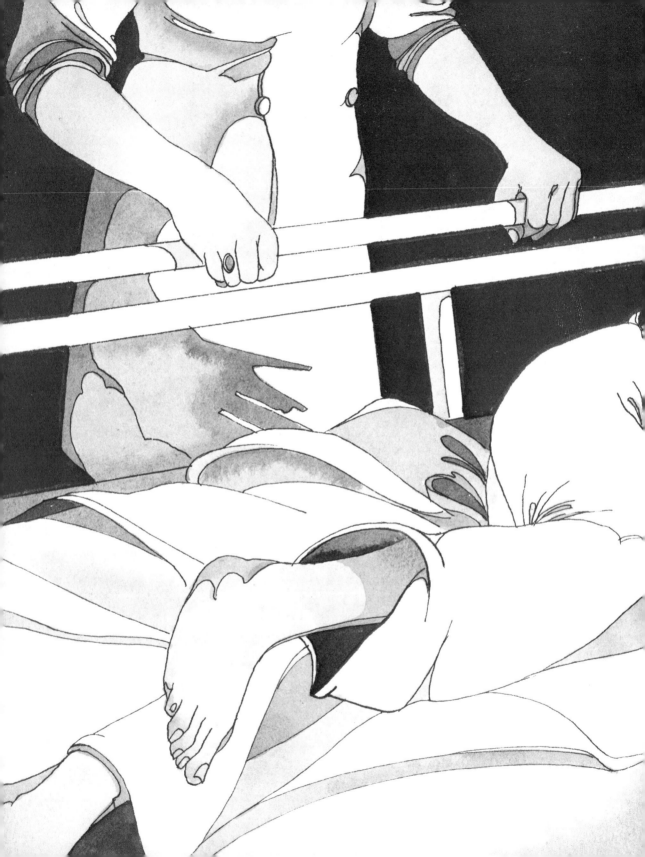

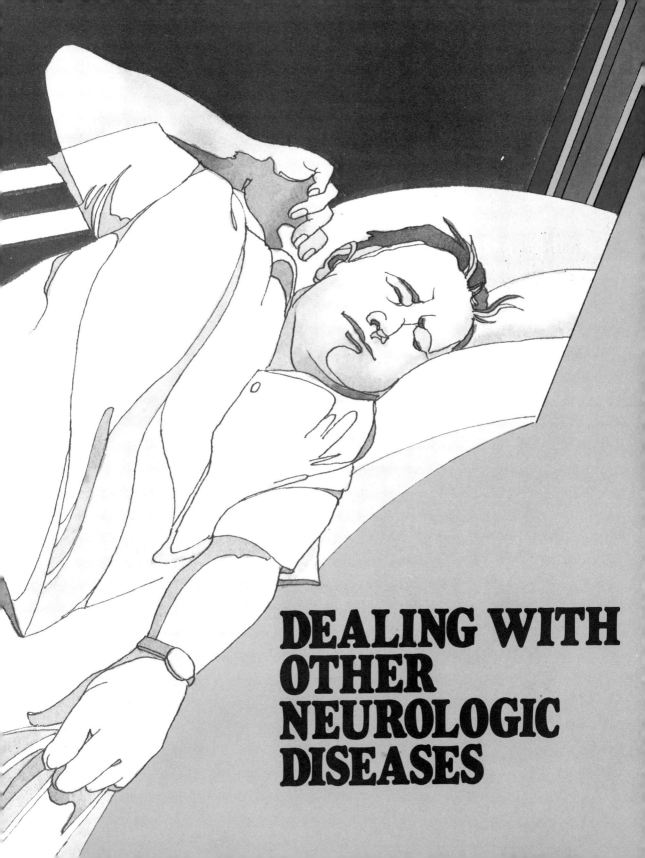

DEALING WITH OTHER NEUROLOGIC DISEASES

During a seizure, what nursing
measures can you take to
protect your patient from injury?

What condition may trigger
a seizure in a patient with a history
of seizure disorders?

What type of seizure is considered an
acute medical emergency?

What two signs signal a meningeal
inflammation?

What Guillain-Barre symptom may be
life-threatening for your patient?

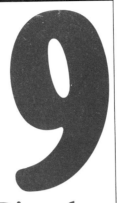

Seizure Disorders
Helping your patient adjust

BY NANCY SWIFT-BANDINI, RN

THE TIME IS LATE AFTERNOON, one hot June day. You've just come on duty in the medical/surgical unit of a small town hospital, when 16-year-old Penny Belden is admitted after suffering a grand mal seizure. According to a girlfiend, Penny had been putting up prom decorations in the high school gym, when suddenly she "started acting funny." Then she fell from the step ladder she'd been standing on and went into violent convulsions, slightly injuring one arm.

When you see Penny, she's already had emergency treatment in the E.D. for her injured arm. However, the nurse was unable to get a complete patient history, because Penny's mother was too upset to answer questions. She kept referring to her daughter's attack as a "fainting spell" and couldn't understand why the doctor wanted to do a complete neurologic workup.

How do you care for a patient like Penny? Do you know what questions to ask those who were present about her seizure? Do you know which tests to prepare her for? And what information to collect for her initial data base?

Suppose the doctor diagnoses Penny as an epileptic? How can you help her if she has another seizure? What must you

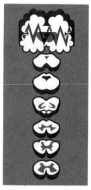

Pathophysiology
Epilepsy is the recurrence of
periodic, excessive, and sudden
outbursts of electrical activity
from abnormal neurons in the
brain causing symptoms that
interfere with normal behavior.
These symptoms we call seizures.
Epilepsy refers only to recurrent
seizures; if the patient suffers a
single seizure, from a head blow,
low blood sugar, fever, or drug or
alcohol withdrawal, he's not an
epileptic.
   Primary epilepsy is the term for
recurrent seizures of unknown
cause.
   Secondary epilepsy is the term
for recurrent seizures from a
known cause: for example, a brain
tumor, trauma, exposure to toxic
substances, prenatal infection,
encephalitis, or meningitis.
   Seizures are also classified
according to their site of origin in
the brain. Those originating from
one specific area are referred to
as *focal* seizures. They usually
affect a single area of the body, as
in a hand tremor or lip smacking.
Seizures that don't have a focal
origin detectable by EEG are
called *nonfocal*.
   You can also describe seizures
a third way — by their clinical
signs. The types of seizures you're
most likely to see are listed on the
opposite page.

teach her about the anticonvulsant medications she'll probably have to take? What should you teach her — and her family
— about her condition?

   If you're not sure how to care for an epileptic patient, you
need to read this chapter. In it, I'll answer all the above
questions — as well as tell you all you need to know about this
complex disease.

Common, but misunderstood

As you probably already know, epilepsy is a common disease.
In fact, it afflicts about one in every 200 Americans. Yet, it's
widely misunderstood by most people, even by some in the
health care field.

   How much do you know about epilepsy? Or about seizures,
which, of course, can occur even in nonepileptic patients. To
check out your understanding of this disease, and update it if
necessary, read the information I've included about seizure
types on the opposite page.

   Remember, however, that some of your patients won't fit
conveniently into these classifications. They may exhibit seizures that deviate from the standard descriptions, or they may
suffer several types of seizures simultaneously.

   Penny, as I mentioned earlier, was admitted to your unit
after suffering a grand mal seizure. But is she epileptic? You
won't know for sure until she's had a complete assessment.

Getting it all together

What's your role in helping the doctor diagnose Penny's condition? Your two main responsibilities are as follows:
   • Tell your patient and her family what tests to expect during
her complete physical and neurologic examination.
   • Collect all the information you'll need about your patient
for a complete data base. Remember, if you didn't witness her
seizure, get an accurate description of it from someone who
did.

   Now let's talk about these responsibilities in more detail. To
start with, what exactly can a patient like Penny expect in a
diagnostic workup? Chances are, the first test the doctor will
order is an electroencephalogram (EEG). The EEG is the
primary diagnostic tool in epilepsy because it helps determine
the location of abnormal electrical discharges in the brain and
may distinguish the type of seizure.

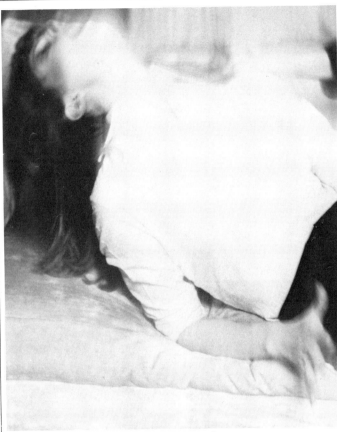

Types of seizures you're likely to see

● *Grand mal* (major motor) seizures always produce a loss of consciousness. Many patients experience an aura or prodrome, such as a change in mood, confusion, blurred vision, or gastrointestinal distress, as the seizure begins.

The seizures produce opisthotonos (arched back) and tonic and clonic movements of all extremities. They may also produce incontinence, frothing at the mouth, and clenching of the jaws. Respiration stops during the tonic phase and may produce cyanosis.

● *Petit mal* (absence attacks) seizures may be inherited and usually occur in children, but in rare cases they occur after age 20. The seizures produce brief periods when the patient appears to be staring or daydreaming, sometimes with rapidly fluttering eyelids. The patient doesn't fall and returns to normal activity without being aware of the attack. He may experience multiple attacks in one day.

● *Myoclonic seizures*, which are also minor motor seizures, are characterized by limb or trunk jerks. (Myoclonus, a normal part of the sleep cycle, is experienced by many people as they fall asleep.)

● *Psychomotor seizures* are sometimes called temporal-lobe seizures because this is the site of origin in many cases. The seizures, which usually occur in adults, may produce automatisms (the repitition of inappropriate acts) such as climbing up and down stairs or pulling off clothing, and are sometimes mistaken for psychotic behavior. Careful observation, and sometimes interviews with a close friend or relative of the patient, are necessary to recognize psychomotor seizures.

● *Jacksonian seizures* usually begin as convulsive movements in one part of the body, such as a trembling hand or foot, and spread to the entire same side of the body. Sensory symptoms include visual, auditory, gustatory, olfactory, and gastrointestinal disturbances. These rare seizures sometimes occur at the onset of grand mal seizures.

● *Status epilepticus* is a series of any type of seizures occurring in rapid succession. (In many cases, status is caused by inadequate anticonvulsant medication.) Status is usually seen with grand mal seizures, is an acute medical emergency, and must be stopped immediately before cerebral hypoxia causes irreversible brain damage.

● *Petit mal status* is less common, but is important because it may be confused with other neurologic dysfunctions. The patient may exhibit amnesia.

● *Psychomotor status,* continuous seizures where the patient repeats inappropriate acts and may even attempt to leave the hospital, is often mistaken for psychotic behavior. Treatment is the same as for petit mal status.

Watch for seizures
Be alert for possible seizures in patients with any of these problems:

TOXIC CONDITIONS
  alcohol withdrawal
  drug withdrawal
  toxins

TRAUMA
  head injuries

NEUROCIRCULATORY
  hemorrhage, e.g., subarachnoid

METABOLIC
  uremia
  diabetes; hypoglycemia
  hypocalcemia
  eclampsia
  fever

INFECTIONS
  meningitis
  brain abscess

NEOPLASMS
  brain tumor
  leukemia

Other tests a seizure patient will probably undergo are a skull X-ray, a computerized axial tomography (CAT scan), and a contrast study to rule out a space-occupying brain tumor. (If you patient is already taking an anticonvulsant for previous seizures, the doctor may also order a check on the serum blood levels for the drug.) To learn how to prepare your patient for these tests, see the Appendices.

Taking the patient's history

Along with the results of these tests, the doctor will need a complete patient history to determine his diagnosis. As you know, a patient like Penny isn't necessarily epileptic because she had a single seizure. Her seizure may have resulted from any one of the many conditions listed on this page.

When you collect data, ask questions that'll help the doctor zero in on the real cause of Penny's seizure. For example, find out if she's had any other accidents, falls, or illnesses that have caused unconsciousness or seizures. Ask if she has a history of alcohol or drug abuse — or if she's inhaled any toxins.

Let's suppose that Penny's mother finally reveals that her daughter has had brief episodes of "daydreaming," when "she just stares and loses track of what's happening." You'd find out all you could about these episodes and document the information carefully. Brief periods of unconsciousness, as you know, suggest petit mal seizures.

Since neither you nor Penny's mother witnessed the grand mal seizure she had at school, you'll have to get the information you need about it from Penny and her girlfriend. When you do, be sure to ask the following questions:

1. Exactly what time — and on what day — did the seizure occur?

2. What was the patient doing just before the attack? Was she excited, sleeping, standing, sitting down? What made you notice the seizure? Did the patient cry out or fall?

3. If the patient has been taking anticonvulsant drugs — Penny wasn't — find out if she's had them on schedule. When was her last dose?

4. How did the seizure develop?

— Was the onset sudden or gradual?

— If the patient's rigidity was superceded by jerks or convulsions, when did this happen?

— What part of the patient's body started moving first?

— Did the convulsions spread? If so, to what parts of the body and in what order?

— Did the patient change body position during the seizure?

— Did she chew, froth at the mouth, roll her eyes?

— If her eyes were open, what did the pupils look like? Did they change in size? Both pupils together, or individually? Did they deviate? If so, to which side?

— How did the patient breathe? In short gasps, slow and evenly, or sporadically?

— How did her skin look? Flushed, ashen, clammy? *Important:* For a short time during a grand mal seizure, a patient normally becomes grossly cyanotic.

— What time did she regain consciousness? Did she fall asleep then? If so, when did she wake up?

— Was the patient incontinent?

5. What was the patient like for about 10 minutes after the seizure? Drowsy? Alert? Active? Did she remember what happened? Were there any injuries?

Be sure to document all the information you gather carefully. Quote the witness exactly in your notes, or write something like "Penny's girlfriend states that 'she seemed to stop breathing, and her face got real dark.'"

In some cases, of course, you'll witness the patient's seizure yourself. If that happens, keep her from injuring herself by following the precautions on page 159. At the same time, observe her condition by using the guidelines I already mentioned and the neurologic assessment in Chapter 2.

Helping your patient stay seizure-free

Eventually, all of Penny's test results are in, and she's had a complete assessment. At that point, the doctor reviews the findings and makes his diagnosis. Penny's EEG shows a non-focal spike and wave pattern, which rules out a focal lesion like a brain tumor. The doctor confirms that she has primary epilepsy, and orders therapy with the following anticonvulsant drugs: phenytoin sodium (Dilantin), 100 mg q.i.d., and phenobarbital 30 mg q.i.d. (see drug chart on page 161).

Although these drugs will not cure Penny's epilepsy, they should keep her seizure-free. Not every patient achieves complete seizure control with medication, however. But in most cases, anticonvulsants significantly reduce seizure severity and frequency.

Danger signals
Any of these conditions in patients with seizure disorders may indicate a serious, perhaps life-threatening, situation:
- Severe injury
- Prolonged apnea; cyanosis
- Cardiac arrhythmias.

DILANTIN (Phenytoin)
PATIENT TEACHING AID

Dear Patient:
Here's what you should know about the drug your doctor has prescribed for you.
Dilantin lessens excessive electrical activity within your brain. This helps to control seizures.
To get the most from your therapy, follow these instructions carefully:

1. You'll probably continue taking this medication for life so you can follow your normal activities. *Don't stop taking your medication,* even if you feel your illness is controlled.

2. Check with your doctor before taking any other medications, including over-the-counter preparations. Inform other doctors you may consult that you're taking this medication.

3. Carry a card stating that you're taking this medication.

4. To minimize redness and overgrowth of your gums, practice good oral hygiene and massage your gums. You may benefit from an electric toothbrush. Visit your dentist regularly.

5. Take your medication with or after meals to reduce the chance of nausea.

6. If you drink alcohol, do so with extreme caution. Alcohol may reduce the effectiveness of your medication.

Call the doctor immediately if you notice any of the following: blurred or double vision, slurred speech, dizziness, headache, unsteady movements or staggering, confusion, skin rash, fever, sore throat, abnormal bleeding, and excessive growth of facial hair. *Inform your doctor at once if you become pregnant.*

One of your responsibilities is to teach Penny — and her family — about the drugs she'll be taking. This is important, because noncompliance with the medication schedule is by far the most frequent reason an epileptic patient suffers recurrent seizures.

In many cases, noncompliance is a form of denial that the patient displays during early drug therapy. This, unfortunately, coincides with the critical period when the doctor must adjust drugs and doses to achieve optimum seizure control.

How can you persuade a patient like Penny to take her medications faithfully? Begin by helping her and her family understand that she will probably have to take anticonvulsant medication for life to remain seizure-free. However, explain that the doctor may initially adjust drugs and doses because the drugs act differently with different people. That will keep her from becoming too discouraged if the anticonvulsants don't immediately control her epilepsy.

Consult with the doctor on Penny's dose scheduling. Why? Because you might learn that the schedule is impractical because two of the doses are scheduled for an hour when Penny

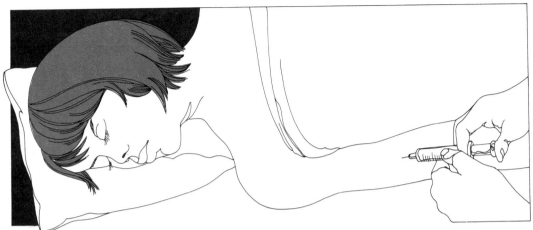

Dealing with a seizure

Suppose Penny, or any other patient, has a seizure while she's in your unit? Here's how you can keep her from injuring herself. (Teach her family these rules, so they can protect her at home.)

1. Remain calm to reassure the patient, if she has not lost consciousness, and other people nearby who may have to assist you.

2. Stay with the patient until the seizure has passed. The convulsions may last only 2 to 5 minutes. If you go for help, the patient may injure herself or choke to death while you're gone.

3. If the patient is out of bed, help her to the floor to prevent her falling. (If the patient has grand mal seizures, the side rails of her bed should be padded and kept in the up position; the bed in the low position.)

4. If the patient hasn't yet clenched her jaws, place something soft, like a folded handkerchief, between her teeth to keep her from biting her tongue. If the patient has dentures, or an orthodontic appliance, try to remove it quickly, but take care not to be bitten. Never force anything between the patient's clenched teeth, lest this cause injury. However, if the patient

moves her jaws in a chewing motion, you may be able to put something between them when her mouth is open.

5. Remove or loosen tight clothing, such as a scarf, tie, or belt.

6. Turn the patient on her side with her head back (hyperextended) and her face slightly downward. This lets secretions and vomitus drain from her airway and lets the tongue fall forward. Some doctors recommend inserting an airway, but only if you've been trained to do so. (In the hospital, a suctioning machine should be kept by the patient's bed to help clear secretions.)

7. Place a small pillow, folded jacket, or other padding under the patient's head, but take care not to flex her neck and obstruct her airway.

8. Don't move the patient, unless she's near something that might cause injury, such as a radiator. Instead, try to move dangerous objects away from the patient. If she's in bed, remove extra pillows and bedclothes which could block her airway. (To avoid this hazard, avoid using pillows to pad side rails.)

9. Don't attempt to restrain the patient during a seizure. This will

usually only make her convulsions more severe and may cause an injury. Her hands can be gently held to prevent their banging. Similarly, a patient wandering around during a temporal-lobe seizure should not be restrained, unless she's in danger.

10. If possible, prevent the patient from becoming a spectacle for curious onlookers. In a hospital, draw the curtain. In a public setting, simply ask bystanders to leave.

11. Reassure and reorient the patient if the seizure has left her frightened or disoriented.

12. If the patient begins to have another attack before regaining consciousness, it may signal the onset of a status epilepticus, a medical emergency. Your first priority is *to support respiration.* Immediately call a doctor, the police, or an ambulance. Stay with the patient, maintain a patent airway, and observe the above precautions until help arrives. In the hospital, anticipate immediate I.V. administration of Valium. Insert an oral airway if possible and suction the patient. The doctor may insert an endotracheal tube and connect the patient to a respirator.

13. Give oxygen after a seizure, if ordered by a doctor.

New surgical procedures

The doctor may decide to try surgery if seizures cause progressively severe brain damage. In any case, he'll consider surgery only after anticonvulsant medications have failed to control seizures.

During the neurologist's and neurosurgeon's initial tests, take care not to give the patient any false hopes for surgical intervention. Surgery may ultimately be contraindicated or, if performed, it may fail to completely control the seizures. However, they may be less frequent and severe.

Advise a patient selected for surgery that he'll be hospitalized for 2 to 6 weeks. If he's on anticonvulsants, the doctor may withdraw them to increase the accuracy of EEG tests used to locate the focus. In some cases, the neurosurgeon will implant depth electrodes through burr holes drilled in the patient's skull, usually over the temporal or frontal lobes. The implanted electrodes are usually left in place for 1 to 3 weeks. During that time, observe the patient carefully for signs of infection or neurologic deficit.

has a class. Ask Penny to describe one of her typical days to you, or refer back to information you gathered for her initial assessment. Then try to find ways that Penny can fit the medication schedule into her routine.

Sometimes a compliance crisis occurs when the anticonvulsant therapy begins to produce good seizure control. For example, a patient like Penny may assume that she is cured because her seizures are controlled. Make sure she and her family don't misunderstand this important point. Warn Penny against overconfidence, so she continues her medication.

Tell Penny ahead of time that she may experience some side effects from the drugs she'll be taking. You can discover what these are by checking the list of anticonvulsants on the opposite page. Then, with the doctor's permission, prepare a patient teaching card about each drug (see the sample on page 158). Go over the information with Penny and her family, so they know what to expect.

Ask about other medications

Before Penny goes home, find out if she takes any other medications that may interact adversely with the anticonvulsants the doctor's ordered. Be sure Penny understands that you're talking about over-the-counter medications, as well as those she may have been given by another doctor. Remind Penny to check with her doctor before she takes any other drugs, and to inform any other doctor or dentist she sees that she's on anticonvulsant therapy,

Also warn Penny and her family to report any sore throat or fever she may have, because it may be an early sign of agranulocytosis. Tell her to inform the doctor about unexplained bruise marks on her skin, because this may be a sign of possible platelet deficiency. Remind her to keep her regularly scheduled doctor's appointments for blood testing and urinalysis.

Helping Penny adjust to her disease

Chances are, Penny will be upset about her disease because of the changes it'll bring in her life. What's more, epilepsy has a stigma attached to it that makes adjustment difficult. One psychiatrist says "the attitude of the public is far more damaging to the epileptic than the disease itself."

You can help Penny face her condition optimistically by

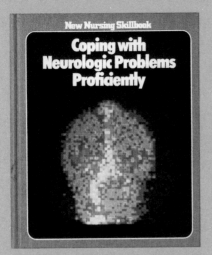
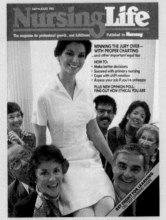

Examine your first—and every volume—free before you buy. Get to know the NEW NURSING SKILLBOOK series...books that help you achieve new proficiency, new confidence.

- Coping With Neurologic Problems Proficiently
- Managing Diabetics Properly
- Monitoring Fluid and Electrolytes Precisely
- Giving Cardiovascular Drugs Safely
- Assessing Vital Functions Accurately
- Nursing Critically Ill Patients Confidently
- Giving Emergency Care Competently
- Reading EKGs Correctly
- Combatting Cardiovascular Diseases Skillfully
- Dealing with Death and Dying

Begin with a 10-day, free examination of *Coping with Neurologic Problems Proficiently.*

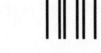
Send this postage-paid card to get your first copy of *NursingLife.*

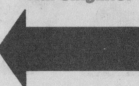

ANTICONVULSANT MEDICATIONS

DRUG	USUAL DOSE	INDICATIONS	TOXIC SIGNS	SIDE EFFECTS
phenobarbital (Luminal)◊	5 to 10 mg/kg/day in children; 30 to 120 mg/day in adults	Grand mal Focal seizures Psychomotor seizures	Nystagmus Ataxia	Sedation Megaloblastic anemia
phenytoin sodium (Dilantin)◊	5 to 10 mg/kg/day in children; 300 to 400 mg/day in adults	Grand mal Focal seizures	Nystagmus Ataxia Lethargy	Gum hyperplasia Megaloblastic anemia
primidone (Mysoline)◊	10 to 20 mg/kg/day in children; 750 mg to 1.5 g/day in adults	Grand mal Focal seizures Psychomotor seizures	Ataxia Nystagmus Lethargy	Sedation Nausea and vomiting
carbamazepine (Tegretol)◊	200 to 400 mg/day in adults, up to 1200 mg/day maximum	Grand mal Focal seizures Psychomotor seizures	Nystagmus Slurred speech Lethargy Nausea and vomiting	Liver toxicity Granulocytopenia Thrombocytopenia
trimethadione (Tridione, Trimedone)◊	300 mg/2 to 3 times a day in children; 600 mg 3 times a day in adults	Petit mal	Sedation Nausea	Acneiform rash Aplastic anemia Blurred vision
ethosuximide (Zarontin)◊	250 mg twice a day in children; 500 mg 4 times a day in adults	Petit mal	Dizziness Nausea and vomiting	Rash Leukopenia
diazepam (Valium)◊	seizure control, 5 to 40 mg/day in adults; status epilepticus, 2 to 5 mg I.V. push q30 minutes until seizures subside	Minor motor seizures Status epilepticus	Lethargy Respiratory depression with intravenous use Ataxia	Rash
clonazepam (Clonopin, Rivotril)◊	0.1 to 0.2 mg/kg/day maintenance dose in children; 20 mg/day maximum in adults	Petit mal Myoclonic seizures	Ataxia Hypersalivation Drowsiness	Behavior changes
valproic acid* (Depakene)	15 mg/kg/day initially; 30 mg/kg/day maximum; (Dose may be increased by 5 to 10 mg/kg/day at 1-week intervals until seizures are controlled, or side effects occur.) If daily dosage exceeds 250 mg, then give in divided doses.	Simple and complex absence seizures including petit mal Adjunctive therapy for mulitple seizure types	Drowsiness Rare hepatic toxicity Rare thrombocytopenia	Nausea and vomiting Diarrhea Transient hair loss

◊Also available in Canada.   *Approved February 1978 by the FDA for use in the United States.

asking what she and her family have heard about epilepsy and then exposing the fallacies. With the doctor's permission, contact the local branch of the Epilepsy Foundation of America (4351 Garden City Drive, Landover, Md. 20781) to provide you with information. Urge Penny to talk about her disease with her doctor, so she can adjust to any new routines without undue difficulty.

Although failure to take anticonvulsant drugs causes most cases of seizure recurrence, other factors can play a part. Warn Penny and her family about these factors. Urge her to avoid extreme physical or emotional stress and disturbing environmental influences (if an EEG shows that they could precipitate a seizure).

Tell her to report any signs of fluid retention, which she may experience before menstruation. And encourage her to eat a balanced diet to avoid nutritional deficiencies. *Nursing tip:* If Penny was of legal age for drinking, you'd also remind her that alcoholic beverages can sometimes precipitate seizures.

Above all, give Penny the reassurance she needs to live with her disease and make a good adjustment to it. You can do this by being sensitive to her feelings and building a rapport, so she'll feel free to ask questions.

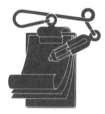

Remember these important points when caring for a patient with a seizure disorder:
1. Be sure to obtain a complete patient history and get an accurate description of the seizure from a witness.
2. Explain to your patient and his family which tests to expect during the physical and neurologic examinations.
3. Consider grand mal, petit mal, myoclonic seizures, status epilepticus, petit mal status, and psychomotor status the most common seizure types.
4. Be alert for seizures in patients with toxic conditions, trauma, neurocirculatory or metabolic problems, and brain infections or neoplasm.
5. Warn your patient about noncompliance with established drug therapy.

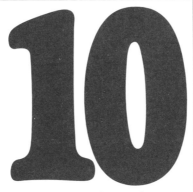

Neurologic Infections
Saving your patient's life

BY SHARON C. SELL, RN

IF YOU'VE STUDIED all the chapters preceding this one, you've read about how to care for patients with most neurologic problems. But what about patients with a neurologic infection; for example, meningitis, encephalitis, or brain abscess? If they're to live, they need prompt, aggressive, medical treatment. They also need the care of a skilled nurse who understands their problems and knows what to do about them.

Are you familiar with the kind of care plan neurologic infections require — and how to implement it? What complications are likely to develop during the disease? How can you prevent them? If you're not certain, you need to read this chapter.

In it, I'll discuss the three infections I mentioned above, as well as the Guillain-Barre syndrome, which may come after infection. Since you'll find the nursing care for meningitis, encephalitis, and brain abscess similar, I'll focus on meningitis. Then I'll tell you how to care for the patient with Guillain-Barre, a frustrating, and sometimes fatal, disorder.

Bob Tucker: A patient with meningitis
Before I get into the case of news reporter Bob Tucker, read the insert on the following page that describes what meningitis

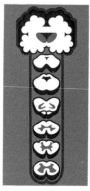

Pathophysiology: Meningitis
Meningitis is an inflammation of the brain and spinal cord meninges. It's usually classified this way:
Acute septic (purulent):
Almost any pathogenic bacteria can cause the disease, but bacteria such as meningococcus, pneumococcus, streptococcus, and hemophilus influenza are usually responsible. Viral forms also occur.

Pathogenic microorganisms may gain access to the meninges and subarachnoid space in these ways: through the bloodstream; after trauma; or from a spreading infection in an adjacent area.
Subacute septic (purulent):
With this type, inflammatory reaction is less severe; onset is less acute; the course of the illness is more prolonged; and relapses are apt to occur. Causes include systemic fungal infections; tuberculosis; syphilis.
Aseptic:
Examination and culture reveal no organisms in the subarachnoid space. The inflammation reaction may be caused by irritants in the subarachnoid space, such as contrast material, drugs, or blood.

is and how it affects the brain. As you may already know, meningitis can be caused by a direct trauma (as it was in Mr. Tucker's case) or a chronic concurrent infection, such as mastoiditis or sinusitis.

To effectively treat meningitis — no matter what its cause — the doctor must first isolate the causative organism in the patient's cerebrospinal fluid (via lumbar puncture), then destroy it with the appropriate antibiotics. If a concurrent infection exists, that must be cleared before treatment for meningitis can be completely effective.

Now let's take a look at 28-year-old Bob Tucker, who walks into the hospital where you work one evening with severe facial injuries. Earlier that evening, he'd been interviewing participants in a massive street demonstration. Then a fight broke out and he got caught in the midst of it.

"I guess I got the worst of it," he says with some difficulty. "I can feel my face swelling up."

You see at once that it's also badly discolored with lacerations of the forehead, nose, and lips. X-rays confirm that he has multiple open fractures of the forehead. These involve the posterior wall of the sinus, which allows access to the brain. However, a neurologic check reveals nothing abnormal, and his vital signs are stable.

Despite Mr. Tucker's protests that "he feels okay," the doctor wants him admitted to the hospital for observation. By noon the next day, Mr. Tucker sees the wisdom of this — for suddenly he "feels terrible and has a severe headache." A quick check of his vital signs reveals that his temperature is 102.2° F. (39° C.), his pulse and blood pressure are elevated, and his respirations are slower.

Besides this, you notice that he's shivering, doesn't respond promptly to normal stimuli, and has nuchal rigidity.

Getting a diagnosis

You immediately call the doctor, who orders a computerized axial tomogram (CAT scan) and lumbar puncture to help him diagnose Mr. Tucker's problem. The results of the CAT scan rule out a cerebral hematoma, but the lumbar puncture shows that Bob Tucker has septic meningitis.

What happens next? First, the doctor will send a specimen of cerebrospinal fluid to the lab for culture, along with specimens of Mr. Tucker's urine, blood, sputum, and

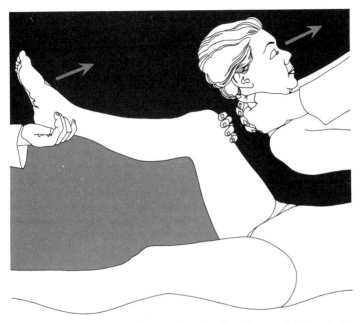

Two signs of meningeal inflammation

BRUDZINSKI'S SIGN
To test for this, place your patient in dorsal recumbent position. Put your hands behind his head and flex his neck forward. Signs of pain or resistance indicate meningeal irritation, neck injury, or arthritis. If he flexes his hips and knees in response to the maneuver, he probably has meningeal inflammation.

KERNIG'S SIGN
To test for this, place your patient in supine position. Flex his leg at the hip and knee, then straighten his knee. Signs of pain or resistance indicate meningeal inflammation.

nasopharyngeal secretions. Then, he'll order antibiotics to be given I.V. (The doctor will also want other routine blood tests taken, including measurement of arterial blood gases to determine possible respiratory problems.)

During this time, of course, you'll continue to assess your patient's condition and take his vital signs. To do this properly, follow the guidelines in Chapter 2, and pay special attention to level of consciousness and cranial nerve involvement. Watch for signs of increasing intracranial pressure, as well as further evidence of increasing meningeal irritation: for example, Kernig's sign and Brudzinski's sign. (To learn how to recognize these last two signs, see above. To review what you've learned about intracranial pressure, read pages 92 to 95.)

What does your ongoing assessment reveal in Mr. Tucker's case? Despite prompt treatment with antibiotics, his condition deteriorates rapidly. Within hours his temperature rises to 105.8° F. (41° C.). He only responds to painful stimuli, and then with nonpurposeful movements.

Understanding your role
Obviously, Mr. Tucker will require truly skilled nursing care just to survive the acute stage of his illness. To insure that he —

Danger signals
Any of these conditions in patients with meningitis may indicate a serious, perhaps life-threatening, situation:
• Elevated temperature above 102.2° F. (39° C).
• Deteriorating level of consciousness
• Onset of seizures
• Altered patterns of respiration.

or any other patient with meningitis — gets this care, the doctor will probably want you to follow these guidelines:
• Continue to administer the antibiotic the doctor has ordered. Make sure you give it *on time* to keep the drug at a therapeutic level in the patient's bloodstream. *Nursing note:* Not all cases of meningitis respond to antibiotics. Sometimes the causative organism is fungal rather than bacterial or viral. For these cases, the doctor will probably choose an antifungal medication such as amphotericin B (Fungizone). If he does, be sure you're familiar with the powerful side effects this drug causes.
• Keep a close watch on the rate and quality of your patient's respirations. Any infection in the brain can cause edema, a hazard to the respiratory center. It may also cause vascular thrombosis of the brain stem. Either of these complications may prove fatal.
• Monitor temperature. If it's elevated, the doctor may want you to give tepid sponge baths, administer antipyretic drugs, or apply ice bags. He may also order a hypothermia blanket. (For tips on how to use a hypothermia blanket properly, see opposite page.)

To help prevent respiratory problems in your patient, turn him at least once every 2 hours, make sure he coughs regularly, and do chest physiotherapy. Have the necessary suctioning, intubation, and oxygen equipment ready in case respiratory distress does occur.

Use the patient's temperature to assess his response to antibiotic therapy and determine the effectiveness of hypothermic measures. If his temperature was low-grade and then suddenly elevates, call the doctor at once. Sudden rise in temperature may mean that the patient is no longer responding to the antibiotic, or the infection requires a different drug.
• Check serum electrolyte measurements regularly to insure proper fluid and electrolyte balance. Keep close track of the patient's intake and output, because dehydration can occur quickly from high fever, decreased level of consciousness, or respiratory problems. If urinary output is inadequate, unexcreted antibiotics may rise to toxic levels in the patient's bloodstream. Check the specific drug he's taking, and note possible side effects. Don't forget to monitor him closely for signs of fluid overload. (This is easier to do if the doctor's ordered a central venous pressure line.)

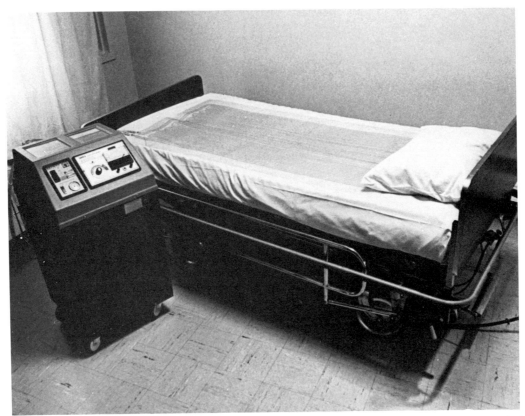

How to manage hypothermia care effectively

When your patient's receiving hypothermia treatments, keep a careful check on his vital signs. Monitor his temperature closely. If he has a rectal probe, check readings every 30 minutes until desired temperature's reached (if no probe, check rectal temperature). Check his blood pressure, pulse, and respirations at least once every half hour until his condition stabilizes. Keep monitoring vital signs periodically after desired temperature's reached.

As you know, shivering is an involuntary muscular activity which occurs in response to cold. It greatly increases metabolism and oxygen requirements. If your patient's shivering, tell the doctor. He may order chlorpromazine (Thorazine) or diazepam (Valium) to control it.

Observe for continued temperature drop. Although some newer units have heating devices to prevent this, others may permit your patient's temperature to drift dangerously low after desired temperature's reached.

If this happens, his level of consciousness may decrease, his reflexes and pupillary responses may diminish, and his urine output may decline. He may even go into ventricular fibrillation or respiratory arrest.

Watch him closely and prevent any extreme drop in temperature.

Take these measures to protect your patient's skin from burns, provide comfort, and facilitate hypothermia:
• Bathe him prior to therapy.
• Apply cold cream or mineral oil to his body.
• Wrap his feet and elbows lightly with Kerlix dressings.
• Don't put layers of sheets, blankets, or sheepskin between your patient and the hypothermia unit. Use only one bath blanket.
• If his doctor says it's okay, turn him every 2 hours. Report any skin discoloration or edema to the doctor.

If the patient must receive an injection, massage and warm the injection site first to help his body absorb the medications.

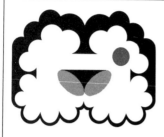

Brain abscess
An abscess within the brain may come from:
• Spreading of an infection of the skull (e.g., otitis, sinusitis, mastoiditis)
• Spreading of an infection between skull and dura (e.g., subdural empyema)
• Direct trauma to the head, allowing entry by pathogenic microorganisms
• Spreading of an infection via the bloodstream, as in bacterial endocarditis.
  Signs and symptoms may include headache, nausea, vomiting, hemiparesis, and seizures. Treatment usually consists of surgical drainage or excision, and antibiotic therapy.

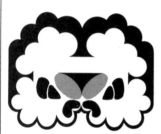

Encephalitis
Encephalitis is an acute inflammatory disease of the brain and meninges, usually caused by a viral infection. The disease may invade the central nervous system via the blood stream or along peripheral or central nerves.
  Some forms, such as St. Louis, Eastern and Western equine, and California, are mosquito-borne. Other forms are carried by ticks.
  Signs and symptoms resemble those of meningitis: headache; nuchal rigidity; deterioration of level of consciousness; cranial nerve abnormalities; and seizures.

• Watch for signs of increased intracranial pressure (see pages 92 to 95). Notify the doctor at once.

• Be alert for possible seizures. For complete information on what to do if your patient has a seizure, see page 159.

• To minimize the irritability and sensitivity to light the infection causes, keep his room darkened and free of unnecessary noise. When he complains of a headache, ask the doctor to order a nonnarcotic analgesic. Applying an ice bag to the patient's head may also help. Log-roll your patient when you turn him, to lessen cervical pain from meningeal irritation.

• Prevent the problems caused by prolonged bedrest by giving your patient good skin care and positioning him properly. For tips on this — as well as exercises to prevent contractures — read pages 64 to 67.

• Try to relieve some of his anxiety and his family's by explaining his disease and its treatment with antibiotics. Keep in mind they'll be particularly upset if the doctor's ordered isolation; for example, with meningococcal meningitis. Listen to their concerns, and get the answers to their questions.

Two other neurologic infections require similar emergency care: encephalitis and brain abscess. What these infections are and how they affect the brain is explained briefly on the opposite page.

Caring for the patient with Guillain-Barre syndrome

Now let's talk about the Guillain-Barre syndrome, an inflammatory disease of the peripheral nervous system (see the explanation on this page). You may not see this disease in many patients but when you do, you'll need to know about it. It can be life-threatening, as well as debilitating. To see your patient safely through it, you'll need: expert nursing skills, innovative procedures, and a warm supportive attitude.

What to expect? Imagine yourself in the neurologic unit of a big city hospital. Back from vacation, you find yourself assigned to care for Matthew Freed, a 34-year-old accountant. According to the report, he's been in the hospital for 10 days. His condition has already been diagnosed as Guillain-Barre syndrome.

From Mr. Freed's history, you see he had a severe upper respiratory infection 3 weeks earlier. Then about 10 days after that, he returned to his doctor complaining of vague malaise, paresthesia and weakness in both lower extremities. He was admitted to the hospital, where the condition was diagnosed. (To confirm the diagnosis, the doctor performed a lumbar puncture, which showed abnormally increased protein and very few white blood cells.) Mr. Freed's symptoms grew steadily worse, until — when you see him — he has flaccid paralysis of his lower extremities.

Will Mr. Freed's condition continue to deteriorate? Well, if he's like many patients with Guillain-Barre, it may stabilize at this point. However, it may also progress up his body toward his head, causing more serious problems. For example, he may develop paralysis of the upper extremities and — even more important — his respiratory muscles. If this happens, the patient's life is in grave danger, and he'll require immediate assisted ventilation. If it progresses upwards still further, Guillain-Barre syndrome may even reach the cranial nerves, affecting their function, or disrupt the autonomic nervous system.

If you've already read earlier chapters, you know what kind of problems Mr. Freed will develop if his disease progresses.

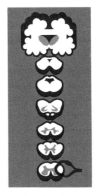

Pathophysiology: Guillain-Barre syndrome

Landry-Guillain-Barre-Strohl syndrome, commonly known as Guillain-Barre, is a demyelinating disease of the peripheral nervous system. Although its precise cause is unknown, it usually occurs after an infection. Anyone may contract Guillain-Barre, regardless of sex or age.

The disease begins as a distal neuropathy and ascends in stages before it stabilizes and gradually starts to resolve itself. Recovery may take up to 24 months, though it may not be complete.

Signs and symptoms may include vague malaise, and a lower extremity weakness that's progressing upward. *Be alert for paralysis of respiratory muscles.*

During this acute stage of his illness, much of the nursing care you'll give him will be the same as described in Chapter 6. However, his prognosis differs from that of a spinal cord-injured patient in this important way: Motor and sensory loss from Guillain-Barre syndrome are seldom permanent. Hopefully, Mr. Freed will recover full functioning when the inflammation from his disease subsides and the myelin sheath regenerates. However, like some patients, he may suffer residual effects. *Nursing tip:* Just as you can expect the paralysis to travel (in an orderly fashion) up his body in the acute state, expect motor and sensory function to return in descending order.

Treating specific problems

As I already mentioned, you'll be caring for Mr. Freed in much the same way as patients with stroke or spinal cord injury. For example, he'll need special attention to prevent respiratory complications — a common cause of death in patients with Guillain-Barre.

To better understand all you need to do, go back and review Chapters 3 and 6. Then we can go on to some of the specific guidelines the doctor will probably want you to follow for a patient like Mr. Freed.

• Relieve the discomfort your patient may feel from abnormal sensations. For example, he may complain of crawly sensations in his mouth or on his arms and legs. Position him comfortably and try leaving his extremities uncovered. Be very gentle when you touch him, as well as when you rearrange bed linen. A mild analgesic may also help.

• Prevent skin breakdown and contractures by giving proper skin care. However, don't permit vigorous exercise because it may increase demyelination. Be sure your patient and his family understand why vigorous exercise is unwise. They may think such exercise will hasten his recover and restore normal functioning.

• Prevent sensory deprivation by talking to your patient every time you enter his room. Explain all procedures and encourage him to ask questions. If your patient seems confused or disoriented, make a special effort to combat this. Get him a calendar with bright colors and bold letters. Ask his family to bring him a clock and a radio. Encourage him to watch television.

• Help your patient communicate. If he has cranial nerve involvement, he may have trouble speaking because his tongue and jaw muscles are affected. Expect his speech to be impaired: for example, slurred, thick, hoarse, or inaudible.

What can you do? If your patient still has motor control in his hands and arms, give him a Magic Slate or a notepad and pencil to communicate with. If he can't use his hands to write, he may be able to use his eyes to communicate by blinking once for "yes" and twice for "no." Make sure he knows that you will check on his needs frequently. If he can use a call cord, keep it within easy reach. Don't be impatient when you have a hard time understanding the patient who can speak. Take time to listen. Your ability to understand may improve with effort. *Nursing tip:* Once you find a way to successfully communicate with your patient, document it on your notes and update his care plan.

• Make sure your patient receives adequate nutrition. Remember, cranial nerve involvement can affect more than his tongue and jaw muscles. It may also affect his gag reflex and make it difficult for him to swallow. Always check your patient's gag reflex before you attempt to feed him. Even if it's intact, it may not be working as well as it should and he will feel like he's strangling. Stay with him for the entire time he's eating. Make sure he doesn't aspirate his food, occluding his airway. Have a suction machine ready, in case of emergency.

To help your patient who's having trouble eating, try these additional suggestions: Allow plenty of time to complete a meal. Avoid drinking straws, which may be hard to manage, and offer a cup or spoon instead. Consult with the dietitian, who can individualize his diet. For example, she may limit the use of milk and milk products since they produce increased mucus. She may eliminate sticky foods like potatoes and spaghetti because they are difficult to swallow. And she may offer thicker fluids because the patient may find them easier to tolerate.

Most Guillain-Barre patients do well on a diet of soft grain foods, fruits, vegetables, and meat purees. If they can't eat, notify the doctor. He may want to order high-calorie, high-protein nasogastric feeding.

Nursing tip: You may want to use a pediatric tube for nasogastric feedings. These tubes are finer and less irritating to

Danger signals
Any of these conditions in patients with Guillain-Barre syndrome may indicate a serious, perhaps life-threatening, situation:
• Deteriorating level of consciousness
• Difficult breathing
• Loss of swallowing and gag reflexes.

the nostrils, so many nurses feel they're less likely to cause fistula formation. However, they do clog easily, so keep feedings very dilute.

Reassure your patient that Guillain-Barre syndrome usually disappears in time and, when it does, he'll regain lost sensory and motor function. Make a special point to mention that this includes sexual function because your patient may be reluctant to ask you about it. Encourage him and his family to talk to you about any fears and worries they may have. When they do, take time to listen. Then be sure to document that the patient needs extra reassurance and support on his care plan.

Hope for a good recovery

As I said at the beginning of this chapter, the patient with meningitis, encephalitis, brain abscess, or Guillain-Barre syndrome needs prompt, aggressive treatment to ensure his chance for recovery. I've outlined what your role as a nurse is in caring for these patients, so you can update your skills. I've also alerted you to some of the complications you may see with these diseases and told you how to help prevent them. Don't forget what you've learned in this chapter. Use these skills to provide better nursing care.

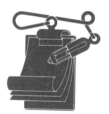

Remember these important points when caring for a patient with a neurologic infection:

1. During your assessment, pay close attention to the patient's level of consciousness and check for cranial nerve involvement.

2. Suspect a meningeal inflammation in a patient with a positive Brudzinski's or Kernig's sign.

3. When using a hypothermia blanket, take care to protect your patient's skin from burns.

3. When your patient's receiving hypothermia treatment, closely monitor his vital signs and temperature.

4. Be aware that Guillain-Barre syndrome usually occurs after an infection and begins as distal neuropathy. Any motor and sensory loss sustained is seldom permanent.

5. If your patient with Guillain-Barre syndrome has trouble communicating, give him a Magic Slate, note pad and pencil, or try devising a system of signals, such as blinking and head nods.

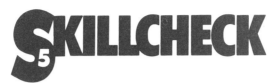

SKILLCHECK

1. You're caring for 45-year-old George McMahon, who's been hospitalized with pneumococcal meningitis. Which of the following is an important nursing measure?
a) Make sure he receives his antibiotic drugs on time.
b) Watch out for the powerful side effects of amphotericin B (Fungizone).
c) Make sure you keep him isolated.
d) Stimulate him every hour with bright lights and loud noises to prevent sensory deprivation.

2. How do you assess a patient for meningeal irritation?
a) Flex one of his legs at the hip and knee and then straighten his knee. Watch for pain or muscle resistance.
b) Stroke the lateral aspect of the sole of your patient's foot. Watch for dorsiflexion of the great toe and spreading of the others.
c) Take his rectal temperature. A temperature over 102° F. (38.9° C.) indicates meningeal irritation.
d) Check for papilledema.

3. When you're caring for Sarah Cranston who has meningitis, you notice changes. She's becoming increasingly lethargic and difficult to arouse. You try to talk to her and discover she doesn't know where she is. What do you do?
a) Call her doctor immediately.
b) Document your findings and continue to observe her.
c) Try to keep her properly stimulated and oriented.
d) Stop giving her the antibiotic the doctor has ordered.

4. Which of the following neurologic infections usually requires postoperative care?
a) Meningitis
b) Encephalitis
c) Brain abscess
d) Rabies.

5. You've just started working in a neurologic unit. The doctor tells you to place one of your patients on a hypothermia blanket to reduce her temperature. As you prepare her for this, which of the following do you do?
a) Place several layers of blankets beneath her to minimize effects of cold.

b) Apply an agent like mineral oil to her skin to protect it from burns.
c) Cover her with several thick blankets to prevent chilling.
d) Warn her not to change position while she's receiving treatment.

6. What's the most serious complication to watch for when you care for a patient with Guillain-Barre syndrome?
a) Paraplegia
b) Seizures
c) Dysarthria
d) Respiratory paralysis.

7. John Barlow has Guillain-Barre syndrome with involvement of his IX and X cranial nerves (glossopharyngeal and vagus). Which of the following problems is he apt to have?
a) Speech difficulties
b) Corneal reflex loss
c) Urinary incontinence
d) Receptive aphasia.

8. You know what causes most recurrent seizures in epileptic patients. How do you use this knowledge when you care for them?
a) Urge each patient to undergo surgery.
b) Teach each patient about the medications he'll be taking.
c) Discourage each school-age patient from participating in extracurricular activities.
d) Refer each patient to a psychiatrist.

9. If your patient has a grand mal seizure while you're caring for him, what do you do first?
a) Run for help.
b) If his teeth are clenched, pry them open with a tongue blade.
c) Turn your patient on his side.
d) Move your patient to a quiet area.

10. Which of these patients is most apt to have a seizure?
a) Patient with asthma
b) Patient with myocardial infarction
c) Patient with peptic ulcer
d) Patient with uremia.

(Answers on page 176)

SKILLCHECK ANSWERS

ANSWERS TO SKILLCHECK 1 (page 49)

Situation 1
d) *Paralysis.* The anterior horn cell bodies are essential if there's to be voluntary and reflex activity of muscles supplied by spinal nerves.

Situation 2
b) *Left hemiparesis or hemiplegia.* The posterior portion of the frontal lobe is responsible for motor activity. Since motor pathways cross as they descend from brain to cord, symptoms will appear on the side of the body opposite the side of the cerebral lesion.

Situation 3
b) *IX glossopharyngeal and X vagus.*

Situation 4
d) *He may have all of the above.* The hypothalamus plays an important role in maintaining bodily homeostasis. It is a thermoregulating center that integrates autonomic activity and controls body water activity.

Situation 5
b) *Tell him that a health-team member will position his head inside a caplike machine. Then he'll take an X-ray and feed the information into a computer to get a more detailed and accurate picture. Reassure your patient that he won't feel any pain.*

Situation 6
d) *Purposeful withdrawal.* Patient can still perceive stimuli and respond appropriately.

Situation 7
c) *Level of consciousness.* A person's conscious level reflects the overall condition of his brain.

Situation 8
b) *Upper motor neuron disease.* This occurs when the plantar reflex is no longer under control of the brain. It indicates that the pyramidal tract is involved.

Situation 9
c) *Pass a wisp of cotton over various areas of his body and note when he feels it.*

ANSWERS TO SKILLCHECK 2 (page 81)

Situation 1
a) *Respiratory.* Airway obstruction or respiratory depression can occur after a stroke and threaten your patient's life. Give it top priority on your assessment checklist.

Situation 2
a) *Corneal abrasion.* When the facial nerve (cranial nerve VII) is affected, your patient can no longer close his eye voluntarily nor will his lacrimal gland supply protective secretions to that eye. Make sure you provide proper eye care.

Situation 3
b) *On his side with his right face uppermost.* This position facilitates drainage and helps prevent aspiration.

Situation 4
d) *His left middle cerebral artery.* Mr. Crane's symptoms, which are right facial paralysis, right hemiplegia, and expressive aphasia, correlate with those expected when brain areas supplied by this artery are damaged.

Situation 5
c) *Symptoms and recovery vary from one patient to another.*

Situation 6
c) *To prevent any arterial blood pressure elevation (which may potentiate rebleeding).* Restrict activity and provide a quiet environment.

Situation 7
b) *Inability to look up or down with the right eye.* An aneurysm on the right internal carotid artery may compress the third cranial nerve (oculomotor) located nearby.

Situation 8
c) *She develops a sudden new headache.* This may indicate a rebleed of the aneurysm or a dangerous rise in intracranial pressure.

Situation 9

a) *To delay clot lysis, which can lead to rebleeding.*

ANSWERS TO SKILLCHECK 3 (page 123)

Situation 1

b) *Realize this is an expected response and anticipate an I.V. order.* Loss of vascular tone below the injury level can cause hypotension and bradycardia.

Situation 2

b) *An automatic bowel and bladder program.* A high thoracic injury spares major respiratory muscles as well as those of upper limbs. Your patient will lose voluntary control of his bowel and bladder but should maintain reflex activity.

Situation 3

a) *Mark it on his skin and inform his doctor.* This indicates progression of spinal cord involvement and may call for immediate treatment.

Situation 4

a) *Tell John that his injury will prevent him from playing basketball.* Be honest with your patient. Don't offer false hope or encourage his denial.

Situation 5

c) *Keep John flat in bed; log-roll him from side to back to side at least once every 2 hours.*

Situation 6

a) *Place her on her side and elevate her head to 30° as ordered.* Elevating her head facilitates venous return, thereby lowering intracranial pressure. Placing the patient on her side will help prevent respiratory problems.

Situation 7

c) *Maintain a sterile system.* The subarachnoid screw allows access to the brain, which increases opportunity for infection. Take precautions to prevent this.

Situation 8

b) *To lower arterial CO_2, which decreases blood volume and therefore ICP.* Hyperventilation helps to eliminate excess CO_2, a potent vasodilator.

ANSWERS TO SKILLCHECK 4 (page 149)

Situation 1

a) *He should lie flat.* This means his head should not be elevated. This position will best facilitate spinal alignment.

Situation 2

c) *Instruct Mr. Nesbitt to remain rigid. Then with assistance turn him as a unit using a pull sheet.* Log-rolling is the best method to maintain spinal alignment while turning the patient.

Situation 3

b) *That he'd probably have to wear a back brace for a while after his surgery.*

Situation 4

b) *If ordered, turn him on his side but keep him flat.* This position facilitates alignment and helps prevent aspiration.

Situation 5

c) *Sensory checks.* This assessment along with motor checks will best indicate improvement or deterioration following Mr. Nesbitt's surgery.

Situation 6

b) *Elevated 30° to prevent an increase in ICP.*

Situation 7

a) *Report it to the doctor at once.* This may be an indication of developing cerebral edema.

Situation 8

c) *Her left pupil remains dilated.* This may be an indication of severely increased ICP.

Situation 9

b) *In a few days, your doctor will probably remove your sutures. Then you can leave your dressing off and wear a wig.*

ANSWERS TO SKILLCHECK 5 (page 173)

Situation 1

a) *Make sure that he receives his antibiotic drugs on time*—the primary means of combating bacterial meningitis. Remember, any disruption in the scheduled dosage time can alter the drug's level in the patient's bloodstream.

Situation 2

a) *Flex one of his legs at the hip and knee and then straighten his knee.* Watch for pain or muscle resistance. This may indicate meningeal irritation and is known as Kernig's sign. Another indication of meningeal irritation is Brudzinski's sign.

Situation 3

a) *Call her doctor immediately.* A deterioration in your

patient's level of consciousness may be your first clue that her brain function is worsening. Prompt treatment is essential.

Situation 4

c) *Brain abscess.* The main treatment for this condition is surgical drainage of the abscess.

Situation 5

b) *Apply an agent like mineral oil to her skin to protect it from burns.* Other measures include turning your patient every 2 hours and applying light Kerlix to her feet and elbows.

Situation 6

d) *Respiratory paralysis.* Ascending motor paralysis may affect the functioning of your patient's respiratory muscles — a life-threatening situation.

Situation 7

a) *Speech difficulties.* These may occur because

motor and sensory portions of the vagus nerve supply the pharynx, soft palate, and larynx.

Situation 8

b) *Teach each patient about his medications.* Remember, noncompliance with his medication schedule is the most frequent reason an epileptic patient suffers recurrent seizures. Assist him to incorporate medication times into his daily schedule.

Situation 9

c) *Turn your patient on his side.* This position allows secretions to drain, and helps keep his airway open. Attempts to restrain or move your patient to another location may injure him.

Situation 10

d) *Patient with uremia.* An increase in metabolic toxins — in this case, urea, may lead to a seizure. Check for an elevation in your patient's blood urea nitrogen (BUN).

ACKNOWLEDGEMENTS

p. 58 Photo courtesy: Milne B. Hewish, Department of Radiology, Temple University Hospital, Philadelphia

p. 101 Chart courtesy: Spinal Injury Nursing Advisory Committee, Rancho Los Amigos Hospital, Downey, Calif.

p. 110 Drawing adapted from material published by Avery Laboratories, Inc., Farmingdale, N.Y.

p. 119 Drawing adapted from material published by Zimmer USA, Warsaw, Ind.

p 185 Photo courtesy: General Electric Company

We gratefully acknowledge the cooperation of the health professionals at Crozer-Chester Medical Center, Chester, Pa., and Doylestown (Pa.) Hospital

Appendices

Common Neurologic Diagnostic Tests

IN THE FOLLOWING PAGES, we'll tell you about some of the most common tests the doctor may use to diagnose your patient's neurologic disease or injury. (Space limitations prevent us from discussing every test.) As you probably know, these tests fall into two categories: invasive and noninvasive.

What's your role when it comes to diagnostic tests? Although you probably won't be with the patient when he undergoes each test, you will need to prepare him for it and care for him afterwards.

What does this entail? The following general guidelines will help you plan care for any patient about to undergo a neurologic test. However, refer to the information we've listed under individual tests for specific details.

Here are the general guidelines:
• Teach your patient all he needs to know about the test. For example, explain what the test is and why it's used, in words he can understand. Tell him what sensations and reactions he can expect to get during the test. Stress the importance of following instructions and staying in the correct position. As you do this, give him a chance to express his fears. Encourage questions so you can clear up any misconceptions.
• Prepare your patient physically. This preparation varies from test to test. Noninvasive tests, such as skull and spinal X-rays, usually require no physical preparation. However, an invasive test such as a cerebral angiogram, requires the following: 1) written permit signed

by patient or appropriate person; 2) baseline vital signs and neurologic assessment; 3) complete restriction of oral intake for specified time; 4) medications, as ordered; 5) removal of prostheses, as well as such items as hairpins and jewelry.

• Understand the risks involved with each test. Watch for signs of complications, but prevent them when possible. Be prepared to cope with any problems that arise.

• Give your patient the care he needs after his test. Observe closely for changes in vital signs and neurologic status. For specific details, read the rest of this section.

Important: Before your patient undergoes any invasive test using a contrast medium, be sure to check if he's allergic to iodine.

Lumbar or cisternal puncture (invasive)

What it is:

Introduction of hollow needle with stylet into subarachnoid space of spinal canal to extract cerebrospinal fluid. Performed under aseptic conditions with applied bactericidal agent. Patient receives local anesthetic. For lumbar puncture (the most common of the two), the doctor inserts needle in vertebral interspace at the L3-4 or L4-5 level. This avoids damage to spinal cord. For cisternal puncture, the doctor inserts needle above the spinous process of C2 vertebra to gain access to the cisterna magna (the space between the cerebellum and medulla).

For either test, the doctor then attaches a stopcock and manometer to the needle to measure the opening pressure of the cerebrospinal fluid. Normal pressure is 50 to 200 mm water. He may perform spinal dynamics to see if there's any fluid blockage. (For complete details on spinal dynamics, see page 142.) He then extracts cerebrospinal fluid samples to check and send to the laboratory for analysis.

Caution: These tests are usually contraindicated for patients with increased intracranial pressure. *Why?* Because the quick reduction in pressure which occurs when fluid is removed may cause brain structures to herniate — leading to death.

What it shows:

Can provide clues to the cause and location of various neurologic problems. The doctor looks for blood, and alterations in appearance, pressure, cell count, and protein content. He may want the fluid cultured to check for organisms.

How to prepare your patient for either test:

Follow general guidelines for invasive tests. Additionally, you should:

• Explain to the patient that he'll feel some pressure pain as the needle's inserted. Caution him not to move suddenly or cough. Tell him to breathe slowly and deeply through his mouth. Explain spinal dynamics, if the doctor plans them (see page 142).

• Before the doctor inserts the needle, position the patient on his side with his knees drawn up to his abdomen and his head bent toward his chest.

Important: You'll probably assist the doctor during this test. If you do, your responsibilities will be as follows: Keep the patient in the proper position; urge him to follow the directions you gave him previously; help the doctor with spinal dynamics, if he plans them; seal collected specimens in sterile containers, label them, and send them to the lab.

How to care for your patient after this test:

Follow general guidelines for invasive tests. If the doctor orders, keep your patient flat for 8 to 10 hours to prevent or minimize headache. Encourage liberal fluid intake. Observe puncture site for redness, swelling, or drainage.

This patient is in proper lateral position for lumbar puncture.

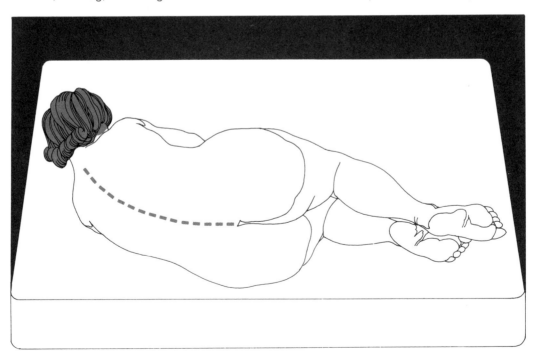

In this CAT scan, the lighter area you see in the left hemisphere indicates an intracerebral hemorrhage. It extends into the basal ganglia and toward the lateral ventricle; the midline is slightly displaced to the right.

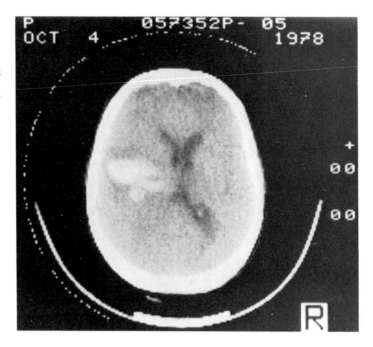

Computerized axial tomography (CAT scan) (invasive or noninvasive)

What it is:
A technique using X-rays (in combination with computer technology) to distinguish between various tissue densities in the brain. Readings are fed into the computer which calculates values and integrates them into composite pictures illustrating brain, bone, and fluid. Shading in these pictures ranges from white (for the most dense tissue) to black (for fluid). Some CAT scans now produce color pictures. If the doctor finds it hard to distinguish between normal and abnormal tissue densities, he may inject a contrast medium.

What it shows:
Reveals tissue densities, so the doctor can check for abnormalities; for example, structural deviations (ventricular enlargement and shifting), and lesions (subdural and intracerebral hematomas, tumors, infarctions, and edema).

How to prepare your patient for this test:
Follow general guidelines. Explain what will happen during the test. For example, tell your patient that he'll lie flat on a table with his head

surrounded by — but not touched by — the machine. Reassure him that this is painless and that the entire procedure lasts approximately 30 minutes. Warn him not to move during the intervals required for each scan. Talking and breathing don't interfere with testing, if he can do them without moving his head.

Nursing tip: Is your patient particularly upset or restless? Tell the doctor. He may want him sedated for the test.

How to care for your patient after this test:
No special care is needed.

Cerebral angiography (invasive)

What it is:
A contrast study, in which a radiopaque dye is injected directly or indirectly into the patient's cerebral circulation. For example, the doctor may inject the dye into one or more of the carotid arteries or, more commonly, he may take an indirect route and inject it into the femoral, brachial, or subclavian arteries.

Serial X-rays are then taken as the dye flows through the vasculature.

A normal cerebral angiogram.

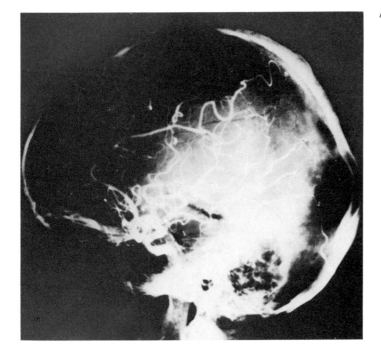

What it shows:
Reveals cerebral circulation, so the doctor can check for structural abnormalities (aneurysms, malformations) and vessel displacement from tumors, hematomas, edema, herniation, and hydrocephalus. He may also use the angiogram to check for abnormal blood-flow patterns caused by arteriovenous malformations, tumors, increased intracranial pressure, insufficient extracranial blood supply, and disrupted collateral circulation. In addition to this, he'll check vessel lumen for patency, narrowing, stenosis, or occlusion.

How to prepare your patient for this test:
Refer to general guidelines for invasive studies.

How to care for your patient after this test:
Follow general guidelines. In addition, do the following: Apply ice to puncture site; observe for swelling, redness, and bleeding; check color, temperature, and pulse of extremity distal to site to make sure blood supply isn't compromised by vasospasm or blood clot.

Besides this, give special care related to the puncture-site's location. If it's in the carotid artery, watch for respiratory distress or arrhythmias. If it's in a subclavian artery, watch for pneumothorax. What about a brachial site? Keep the patient's arm immobilized and don't take his blood pressure in that arm. Immobilize the patient's leg for puncture site in a femoral artery.

If bleeding occurs, apply manual pressure.

This spinal X-ray indicates a fracture of the 12th thoracic vertebra.

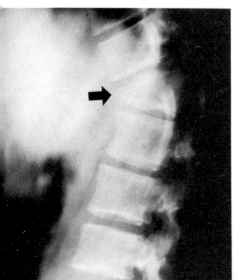

Skull or spinal X-ray (noninvasive)

What it is:
Flat plate and/or tomogram.

What it shows:
Reveals patient's bony structures, so doctor can check for abnormalities; for example, deformities, calcifications, or altered bone densities.

How to prepare your patient for this test:
No special physical preparation needed. Follow general guidelines.

How to care for your patient after this test:
No special care needed.

Brain scan (invasive)

What it is:
A technique in which a small amount of radioisotope is injected intravenously. The gamma rays produced are then measured by a special scanning instrument.

What it shows:
Reveals uptake and distribution of isotope in the brain, so doctor can check for abnormalities. A positive scan (showing increased focal uptake) may indicate tumor, subdural hematoma, abscess, or infarct. A negative scan doesn't necessarily rule out an intracranial lesion, but may serve as a baseline if later problems arise.

How to prepare your patient for this test:
Follow general guidelines for invasive tests. Tell him that the procedure takes only a few minutes.

How to care for your patient after this test.
No special care needed. Follow general guidelines.

The patient shown below is undergoing a brain scan.

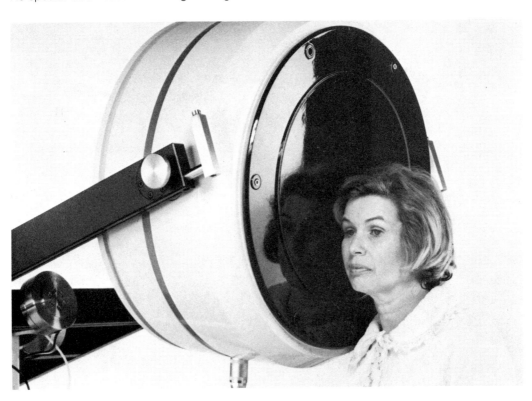

Electroencephalogram (noninvasive)

What it is:
Reveals brain wave patterns, so doctor can check for abnormalities. He may use this test to detect epilepsy or other convulsive disorders; to help determine cause of stupor or coma; to help locate surface brain lesions; to monitor course of neurologic disease or injury; to monitor cerebral function during anesthesia; and to help determine medical brain death.

How to prepare your patient for this test:
Follow general guidelines. Additionally, wash the patient's scalp and hair before electrodes are attached. Make sure he avoids coffee, tea, and other stimulants. Encourage him to ask questions about the test, so you can clear up any misconceptions he may have. For example, you have to reassure him that he won't receive an electric shock.

How to care for your patient after this test:
You'll have to wash the patient's scalp and hair to remove residual paste. Other than that, no special care is needed.

Myelogram (invasive)

What it is:
A contrast study, in which a contrast medium (dye or air) is injected into the spinal subarachnoid space and/or the cisternum magnum. The doctor can then visualize the patient's spinal column and underlying structures via fluroscopy. X-rays can be taken of selected areas.

What it shows:
Reveals patient's spinal subarachnoid space, so doctor can check for abnormalities; for example, bony changes, partial or complete obstruction of subarachnoid space, congenital lesions, spinal cord compression and displacement.

How to prepare your patient for this test:
Follow general guidelines for invasive tests. In addition, warn your patient that he may feel some discomfort during the procedure, but that he'll receive a local anesthetic. Tell him that he'll be tilted up and down on a special table during the test. Encourage him to ask questions, so you can clear up misconceptions.

How to care for your patient after this test:

Refer to the care given to patients after a lumbar or cisternal puncture. Ask the doctor if he has any special instructions for positioning the patient's head. These may vary, depending on the contrast medium used. Report any complications your patient may have after this test: for example, stiff neck, temperature elevation, headache, and urinary retention.

Cerebral-evoked potentials (noninvasive)

What it is:

A technique using three different testing procedures that detects, records, and amplifies cerebral electrical potentials generated from a series of stimuli using electrodes. The testing procedures include: brain stem auditory-evoked potentials (BAEP); somatosensory-evoked potentials (SEP); and visual-evoked responses (VER).

What it shows:

Reveals brain wave amplitudes and patterns so the doctor can check for any abnormalities: for example, schwannomas;

In this photo, the patient is undergoing a myelogram.

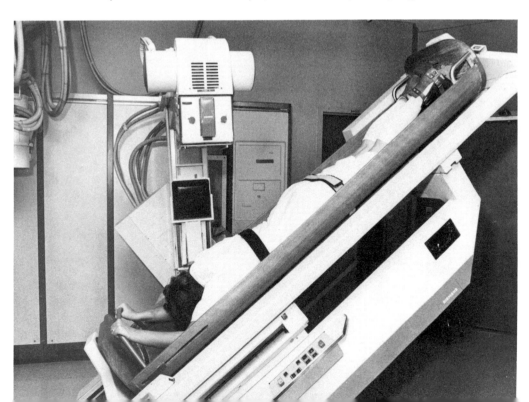

optic nerve neuropathies; and spinal myelopathies. The BAEP, SEP, and VER procedures help the doctor identify and evaluate pathologies that may not be detected by computerized axial tomography (CAT), arteriography, or myelography.

How to prepare your patient for this test:
Follow general guidelines for noninvasive tests. Because this test doesn't require patient cooperation, uncooperative patients may receive sedation without significantly affecting test result.

How to care for your patient after this test:
Depending on electrode placement, you may have to wash the patient's scalp and hair or limbs to remove residual paste. Other than that, no special care is needed.

NURSES' GUIDE TO
Chronic Neurologic Problems

AS YOU KNOW, this Skillbook focuses on the nursing care you'll give to patients suffering from acute neurologic diseases and injuries. However, we know that you may also care for patients with the following chronic neurologic problems: Parkinson's disease, multiple sclerosis, amyotrophic lateral sclerosis, Huntington's chorea, and myasthenia gravis. For this reason, we've included the following brief, but helpful, reference charts to bring you up to date.

Today, no cure exists for any of these problems. However, the efforts of dedicated researchers have contributed much to our understanding and care in this area. Medications have provided effective symptomatic relief for patients with myasthenia gravis and, recently, for patients with Parkinson's disease. We are hopeful that other treatments will be discovered for the remaining chronic neurologic problems—with an eventual cure for all.

Most patients victimized by these devastating problems are cared for at home, in a clinic, or in a long-term care facility. However, you may see some in a general hospital setting if their conditions become acute. Hopefully, the following reference charts will give you some idea of what to expect.

NURSES' GUIDE TO CHRONIC NEUROLOGIC PROBLEMS

HUNTINGTON'S CHOREA

PATHOLOGY	DIAGNOSIS	CAUSE	AGE GROUP; SEX
	No known test to confirm diagnosis. Usually determined by history and physical.	Exact cause unknown; however it's a hereditary disease transmitted through a dominant autosomal gene. Can be transmitted by either sex; can be inherited by either sex. Each offspring has a 50% chance of inheriting the disease.	Onset: Usually ages 35 to 50. Affects both sexes.

An extrapyramidal syndrome characterized by degeneration in caudate nucleus and putamen of basal ganglia.

MULTIPLE SCLEROSIS

PATHOLOGY	DIAGNOSIS	CAUSE	AGE GROUP; SEX
	Examination of cerebrospinal fluid shows an increase in gamma globulin fraction on protein electrophoresis.	Exact cause unknown, though some doctors suspect virus or abnormal immune response. Note: MS occurs mainly in cold, damp climates.	Onset: Usually ages 30 to 35. Affects more females than males.

Plaques or patches of demyelination scattered throughout CNS.

SIGNS AND SYMPTOMS	TREATMENT	NURSING CARE
Choreiform movements and dementia: • Very rapid, purposeless movements, often violent. • Facial grimacing, tongue-smacking • Dysarthria • Severe personality change • Patient eventually becomes totally dependent. Death usually occurs in 10 to 15 years, sometimes from suicide; sometimes from congestive heart failure or pneumonia.	No known treatment to cure or alter course of disease. Symptomatic treatment only. Medications used with minimal success: • chlordiazepoxide (Librium) • haloperidol (Haldol) • chlorpromazine (Thorazine) • imipramine (Tofranil).	Physical and emotional support: • Explain disease • Provide basic needs: hygiene, skin care, bowel, bladder care. Also, adequate nutrition and suicide precautions. Refer patient and family to: • Committee to Combat Huntington's Disease (CCHD) • Visiting nurse service • Social service • Genetic counseling • Long-term care facility, if needed.

SIGNS AND SYMPTOMS	TREATMENT	NURSING CARE
Disease course lengthy; marked by remissions and exacerbations: • Visual problems (nystagmus, diplopia, and field-cuts) • Slowing and slurring of speech • Muscular weakness • Poor coordination • Paresthesias • Inappropriate emotional responses • Bowel and bladder dysfunction. Secondary problems include urinary tract infections, nutritional disturbances, emotional upsets, joint contractures, crippling.	No known treatment to cure or alter course of disease. Symptomatic treatment only. Medications may include: • dantrolene sodium (Dantrium), diazepam (Valium), to reduce spasticity • steroids: I.V. ACTH or oral prednisone. Used only during exacerbation to reduce inflammation in demyelinated areas. Patient may also receive occupational therapy to improve daily living activities, and physical therapy for gait problems and spasticity.	Help patient set realistic goals. Teach patient about: • His disease • Proper nutrition and rest • Self catheterization, if doctor orders intermittent catheterization • Alternate patching of eyes, if he has diplopia. Refer to: • Social service • Physical therapy • Visiting nurse service • Homemakers service • Multiple Sclerosis Society.

NURSES' GUIDE TO CHRONIC NEUROLOGIC PROBLEMS

AMYOTROPHIC LATERAL SCLEROSIS

PATHOLOGY	DIAGNOSIS	CAUSE	AGE GROUP; SEX
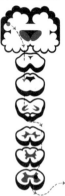 Progressive disorder affecting both upper and lower motor neuron systems. Characterized by atrophy of motor (Betz) cells in corticospinal tracts.	No known test to confirm diagnosis. Usually determined by history and physical and by ruling out other neurologic problems.	Exact cause unknown, though some doctors suspect Vitamin E deficiency, virus, or abnormal immune response.	Onset: Usually ages 50-80 Affects more males than females.

PARKINSON'S DISEASE

PATHOLOGY	DIAGNOSIS	CAUSE	AGE GROUP; SEX
 An extrapyramidal disorder affecting the basal ganglia; related to dopamine deficiency.	No known test to confirm diagnosis. Usually determined by history and physical, and by ruling out other neurologic problems.	Exact cause unknown, although dopamine deficiency proven. Parkinsonian symptoms have been linked to: • Arteriosclerosis • Encephalitis • Carbon monoxide, mercury, manganese poisoning • Midbrain compression.	Onset: Usually ages 60 to 80. Affects more males than females.

SIGNS AND SYMPTOMS	TREATMENT	NURSING CARE
Vary depending on which motor cells are affected. Starts with: • Irregular twitchings in affected muscles. • Muscular weakness Progresses to: • Muscular atrophy and eventual paralysis. Patient becomes totally dependent. *Note:* No sensory or mental deficits. Usually fatal in 3 to 20 years.	No known treatment to cure or alter course of disease. Symptomatic treatment only. • Antibiotics for respiratory or urinary infections. • Tracheostomy with ventilatory assistance for respiratory paralysis.	Teach patient about disease. Provide good skin care, adequate nutrition (possibly tube feedings), and emotional support. Help patient communicate. Assist in positioning and transferring. Refer patient and family to: National Association for Amyotrophic Lateral Sclerosis.

SIGNS AND SYMPTOMS	TREATMENT	NURSING CARE
Characterized by rigidity, slowing of movements, and involuntary tremor. Patient shows: • Difficulty chewing, swallowing • Tremor beginning in upper limbs. Can progress to lower limbs. • Slowness of movements. • Initial rigidity in arms, resulting in jerky "cogwheel" motions; later rigidity can affect all joints, causing painful contractures • Locomotion problems; slow, shuffling gait with loss of arm swing. Patients sometimes build up speed and must be stopped in order to slow down. • Mask-like, staring face • Body held in moderate flexion • Excessive sweating and salivation.	No known treatment to cure disease. Medications: Those containing L-dopa have drastically improved symptoms, as well as prognosis of many patients. • levodopa (Larodopa) • carbodopa/levodopa (Sinemet). Physical therapy: exercises to reduce rigidity. Surgery: For some patients, stereotaxic measures to destroy parts of the thalamus.	Teach the patient about: • His disease • His medications (Assist in drug regulation period — observe for potent side effects as well as desired responses.) Provide supportive care: • Adequate nutrition. Encourage patient to eat semisolid food, if he has difficulty in chewing or swallowing. • Emotional support. • Physical therapy, as ordered. • Stress need for continued checkups. Refer patient to: • Physical therapist • Visiting nurse, if needed.

NURSES' GUIDE TO CHRONIC NEUROLOGIC PROBLEMS

MYASTHENIA GRAVIS

PATHOLOGY

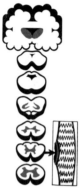

Thought to be deficiency of the chemical, acetylcholine. (This chemical facilitates passage of motor impulses from nerve terminals to skeletal muscle fibers.)

DIAGNOSIS

Doctor gives 2.5 mg of neostigmine methylsulfate with 1/100 gr of atropine sulfate by subcutaneous injection. If the patient has myasthenia, her muscle activity will return to normal within 45 minutes and the effect will last several hours.

Or, doctor gives up to 10 mg tensilon, I.V., but the effect lasts only 5 to 10 minutes.

CAUSE

Exact cause unknown, though some doctors suspect a relationship between immune mechanism originating in the thymus gland and the chemical reactions at the neuromuscular junction.

AGE GROUP; SEX

Onset: Usually ages 20 to 50.

Affects more females than males.

SIGNS AND SYMPTOMS

Abnormal muscular fatigue, evidenced by progressive weakness of muscles as patient uses them.

Symptoms include:
- Bilateral ptosis of the eyelids
- Blurred or double vision
- Impaired swallowing
- Voice weakness
- Difficulty maintaining head position
- Generalized muscular weakness when other muscle groups are affected.

Myasthenic crisis occurs when weakness of respiratory muscles produces acute respiratory failure.

Cholinergic crisis occurs when too much anticholinesterase medication causes respiratory failure. To distinguish the difference, the doctor gives tensilon. If the patient improves, it was a myasthenic crisis; if she gets worse, it was a cholinergic crisis.

TREATMENT

No known treatment to cure disease.

Medications include:
- pyridostigmin bromide (Mestinon)
- neostigmine (Prostigmin)
- ambenonium (Mytelase)

The above drugs inhibit cholinesterase activity which is thought to break down acetylcholine. Taken regularly, for life, they're effective in relieving symptoms.

The doctor may also order steroids. When severe symptoms exist, these may be used to block immune mechanism and restore chemical reaction at the myoneural junction.

Surgery: For some patients, thymectomy

If indicated, the doctor will perform a tracheostomy, or intubate the patient.

NURSING CARE

- Teach the patient about her medications and disease.
- Refer her to Myasthenia Gravis Foundation
- Urge her to report new symptoms to doctor.
- Help her plan daily activities to correspond with strength; tell her to avoid physical and emotional stress.
- Explain eye patching for diplopia
- Provide good respiratory care during myasthenic or cholinergic crisis.

Glossary

acetylcholine — the chemical substance active in nerve impulse conduction across nerve synapses and myoneural junctions.

agranulocytosis — an acute condition, found mostly in drug sensitization cases; characterized by sudden drop in leukocyte production making the body susceptible to bacterial invasion.

aphasia — inability in any phase of understanding or using spoken and written language. Words are heard in the temporal lobe and seen in the parieto-occipital area; expressive speaking comes from the inferior-posterior frontal area, and writing from the posterior frontal area.

arachnoid mater — see *Meninges*.

atherosclerosis — narrowing of the lumen of arterial walls from fatty plaque accumulation.

cerebellum — the small, fine-textured distinct lobes of the brain sitting below and in back of the cerebrum, the brain's largest part; the cerebellum is concerned with coordinating movements.

cerebrum — in man, the brain's main portion; the two cerebral hemispheres are united by a thick bundle of nerve fibers, the corpus callosum. Contains the frontal lobes in the forehead, the temporal lobes under the temples, the parietal lobes at the crown of the head, and the occipital lobes in back.

clonic — rapid muscular spasms in which there's alternate contraction and relaxation.

conjugate gaze — a normal state, in which both eyes look in the same direction at the same time. Coordinated, working in unison.

contractures — shortening of muscles from disuse, which makes them resistant to stretching and leads to deformity.

contralateral — in, on, or pertaining to the opposite side.

convulsion — paroxysms of involuntary muscular contraction and relaxation.

cortex — an outer layer. The cerebral cortex is the convoluted layer of gray matter that covers the cerebral hemispheres, about half of it hidden within the deep grooves, or sulci, folded within the elevations, or gyri.

cranial nerves — the 12 pair of nerves contained in the skull as opposed to the spinal cord; they control the five senses, plus eye, mouth and facial movement and sensation, mastication, and swallowing.

decerebrate — abnormal posture occurring in the unconscious patient in which patient's upper and lower limbs usually are rigidly extended. Indicates cerebral damage usually from brain-stem injury.

decorticate — abnormal posture occurring in the unconscious patient; indicates cerebral damage from which the patient's upper limbs usually are flexed and his lower limbs are extended.

demyelination — removal or destruction of myelin nerve covering.

dura mater — see *Meninges*.

dysphasia — diminished ability to understand or express written or spoken language.

dysrhythmia — disturbance of normal rhythm such as abnormalities in brain waves, as recorded by encephalography.

epidural — outside the dura.

flaccid — loss of muscular tone resulting in limp, flabby appearance.

grand mal — a type of epileptic seizure with convulsions and loss of consciousness.

hemianopsia — blindness involving one-half of the visual field. Types are: homonymous — involves right or left half of the visual field in each eye; bitemporal — involves the temporal half of the visual field in each eye; binasal — involving the nasal (medial) half of visual field in each eye.

hemiparesis — muscular weakness on one side of body only.

hemiplegia — muscle paralysis on one side of the body only.

hyperesthesia — increased sensitivity to pain and touch stimuli.

hyperextend — to extend limb or body part beyond its normal limit.

hypothalamus — nuclei of gray matter in the base of the brain under the thalamus, and connected with the pituitary. It regulates many functions including visceral activities, water balance, temperature, and (in association with the reticular formation) sleep.

incontinence — inability to control defecation and urination.

intracerebellar — occurring within the cerebellum, or inferior part of brain.

ipsilateral — pertaining to same side of body; homolateral.

laminectomy — surgical procedure in which laminae of one or more vertebrae are removed.

lysis, lytic — breaking down or releasing of a chemical substance in the process of dissolution or disintegration.

mastoiditis — mastoid process inflammation of temporal bone.

medulla oblongata — part of the brain stem just below the pons and joined to the spinal cord. Numerous cranial nerves originate here. Plays role in regulating heart, blood pressure, and breathing.

meninges — membranes covering the brain and spinal cord: 1) dura mater — the outermost, toughest, and most fibrous of the three membranes; 2) arachnoid mater — the middle membrane: A fine, delicate structure that conforms to the pia mater but is separated from it by the subarachnoid space; 3) pia mater — the innermost membrane containing the vascular network: a fine areolar tissue, which follows the fissures and contours of the brain.

myelinated — refers to nerves protected with a white, fatty coating: the myelin sheath.

myoclonic — spasms or twitching of a muscle or group of muscles.

neuron — the nerve cell, including a cell body, dendrites (branches conducting impulses to the cell body), and an axon (the single fiber conducting impulses away from the cell body).

nuchal rigidity — denotes meningeal irritation with neck stiffness and resistance to passive movements.

nystagmus — an oscillating eyeball movement; involuntary and repetitive.

oscillation — a rhythmic, pendulum-like movement; vibration or tremor.

paresis — muscular weakness from brain and/or spinal cord involvement.

paresthesias — abnormal skin sensations: for example burning, numbness, and tingling.

petit mal — a mild, nonconvulsive, epileptic attack with momentary loss of consciousness.

phrenic nerve — this nerve, which activates respirations, originates in the cervical plexus of the spinal cord and extends through the thorax to the diaphragm. It causes diaphragm to contract, starting the inspiration process.

pia mater — see *Meninges*.

pons — part of the brain between the midbrain and the medulla; seen as a bulge at the top of the brain stem.

proprioceptive — describes a patient's awareness of the minuscule adjustments in equilibrium necessary for the maintenance of his posture, balance, and position changes.

ptosis — drooping, as of the upper eyelid from third cranial nerve paralysis.

pulmonary embolism — the sudden occlusion of a lung artery or arterial branch by a foreign substance or blood clot.

reticular activating mechanism — the alerting system of the brain. Extends from central brain stem area to all parts of cerebral cortex. It initiates and maintains wakefulness, introspection, and attention.

seizure — convulsion or attack of sudden, unpredictable onset.

sensory deprivation — lack of satisfactory interaction with one's own environment causing faulty memory and impaired reasoning.

septic — condition resulting when bacterial infection produces toxic substances and causes tissue deterioration.

serosanguineous — discharge or exudate composed of both blood and serum.

sinusitis — inflammation of the nasal sinus cavities.

spastic — abnormally increased muscle tone.

stimulus — anything capable of eliciting a response such as muscular contraction, gland secretion, or nerve impulses, from a living organism.

subarachnoid space — the area between the arachnoid mater and the pia mater which contains cerebrospinal fluid.

supraorbital — located above bony socket area of eyeballs.

synapse — the space between the axon of one nerve cell and the dendrite of another, across which nerve impulses are conducted. This synapse is polarized, allowing nerve impulses to be transmitted in one direction only.

tactile — sense of touch; ability to feel.

thrombophlebitis — clot development from inflammatory changes in venous walls.

tinnitus — abnormal noises heard in the internal ear; for example, ringing, buzzing.

tonic — prolonged muscular contraction or tension.

vasospasm — blood vessel spasm causing narrowing of the lumen.

visceral — pertains to internal body organs in abdomino-pelvic and thoracic regions.

Index

Selected References

Blout, M., et al. "Symposium on Care of the Patient with Neuromuscular Disease: Management of the Patient with Amyotrophic Lateral Sclerosis," *Nursing Clinics of North America* 14: 157-171, March 1979.

Bydder, G.M., et al. "Clinical NMR Imaging of the Brain: 140 Cases," *American Journal of Radiology* 139:215-236, August 1982.

Chusid, Joseph G. *Correlative Neuroanatomy and Functional Neurology,* 17th ed. Los Altos, Calif.: Lange Medical Publications, 1979.

Conway, Barbara Lang. *Carini and Owens' Neurological and Neurosurgical Nursing,* 7th ed. St. Louis: C.V. Mosby Co., 1978.

Coping With Neurologic Disorders. Nursing Photobook™ Series. Springhouse, Pa.: Springhouse Corporation, 1981.

Davis, Joan E., and Mason, Celestine B. *Neurologic Critical Care.* New York: Van Nostrand Reinhold Co., 1979.

Dunsker, Steward. "Lumbar Disc Disease—Diagnostic and Therapeutic Aspects," *Contemporary Neurosurgery* 4(8), July 1982.

Green, Barth, et al. "Kinetic Nursing for Acute Spinal Cord Injury Patients," *Paraplegia* 18:181-186, 1980.

Heiden, James, and Weiss, Martin. "Management of Cervical Spinal Cord Trauma in Southern California," *Journal of Neurosurgery* 43:732-736, 1975.

Hickey, Joanne. *The Clinical Practice of Neurological and Neurosurgical Nursing.* New York: J.B. Lippincott Co., 1981.

Jones, Cathy, and Cayard, Carol. "Care of ICP Monitoring Devices: A Nursing Responsibility," *Journal of Neurosurgical Nursing* 14(5): 255-261, 1982.

Litel, Gerald R. *Neurosurgery and the Clinical Team: A Guide for Nurses, Technicians, and Students.* New York: Springer Publishing Co., 1980.

Merritt, H. Houston, ed. *A Textbook of Neurology,* 6th ed. Philadelphia: Lea and Febiger, 1979.

Nudleman, Kenneth, and Kusske, John. "Evoked Potentials in Neurosurgical Practice," *Contemporary Neurosurgery* 3(26), March 1982.

Omer, George E., and Spinner, Morton. *Management of Peripheral Nerve Problems.* Philadelphia: W.B. Saunders Co., 1980.

Patten, John. *Neurosurgical Differential Diagnosis.* New York: Springer-Verlag, 1980.

Plum, Fred, and Posner, Jerome. *The Diagnosis of Stupor and Coma,* 3rd ed. Philadelphia: F.A. Davis Co., 1980.

Suchenwirth, Richard. *Pocket Book of Clinical Neurology,* 2nd ed. Chicago: Year Book Medical Publishers, Inc., 1979.

Sunderland, Sydney. *Nerves and Nerve Injuries,* 2nd ed. New York: Churchill-Livingston, Inc., 1979.

Swift-Bandini, Nancy, and Mabel, Robert M. *Manual of Neurological Nursing.* Boston: Little, Brown & Co., 1978.

Taylor, Joyce, and Ballenger, Sally. *Neurological Dysfunction and Nursing Interventions.* New York: McGraw-Hill Book Co., 1980.

Tindall, George, et al. "Neurosurgery — The Year in Review – 1981," *Contemporary Neurosurgery* 3(27), 1982.

Youmans, Julian R. *Neurological Surgery: A Comprehensive Reference Guide to the Diagnosis and Management of Neurosurgical Problems,* 2nd ed. Philadelphia: W.B. Saunders, 1982.